Addicted to Rehab

CRITICAL ISSUES IN CRIME AND SOCIETY

Raymond J. Michalowski, Series Editor

Critical Issues in Crime and Society is oriented toward critical analysis of contemporary problems in crime and justice. The series is open to a broad range of topics including specific types of crime; wrongful behavior by economically or politically powerful actors; controversies over justice system practices; and issues related to the intersection of identity, crime, and justice. It is committed to offering thoughtful works that will be accessible to scholars and professional criminologists, general readers, and students.

For a list of titles in the series, see the last page of the book.

Addicted to Rehab

RACE, GENDER, AND DRUGS IN THE ERA OF MASS INCARCERATION

ALLISON McKIM

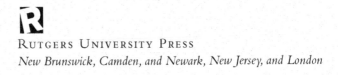

RUTGERS UNIVERSITY PRESS
New Brunswick, Camden, and Newark, New Jersey, and London

978-0-8135-8762-2
978-0-8135-8763-9
978-0-8135-8764-6
978-0-8135-8765-3

Cataloging-in-Publication data is available from the Library of Congress.

A British Cataloging-in-Publication record for this book is available from the British Library.

∞ The paper used in this publication meets the requirements of the American National Standard for Information Sciences—Permanence of Paper for Printed Library Materials, ANSI Z39.48–1992.

www.rutgersuniversitypress.org

Manufactured in the United States of America

*I dedicate this book to the women in my life:
my mother, sister, and friends. I depend on you.*

Contents

Addicted to Rehab

Introduction

REHAB IS THE NEW BLACK

CHRISTINE WAS IN REHAB when she decided to have an abortion. A court had sentenced Christine to a year of addiction treatment at a program called Women's Treatment Services (WTS) instead of sending her to prison.[1] Funded by the state's criminal justice system, WTS is one of many nonprofit agencies that provide mandated addiction treatment as an alternative to incarceration. Reformers and officials hope that such treatment will end mass incarceration, reduce recidivism, and save money. But WTS has additional goals: it seeks to challenge race and gender injustice by "empowering" its clients with what it calls "women-centered" treatment. Christine was a reserved woman in her twenties, and like most of the women in WTS and the state's prisons, she was African American and came from a low-income background. I heard her announce her decision to have an abortion while I was observing WTS's weekly parenting class. WTS's family counselor, Karen, pushed the women to discuss their feelings of guilt and shame about their failures as mothers. Karen emphasized that they had to "process" these emotions before they would be ready to leave.

When Christine shared her decision with the group, she explained that she had ended the pregnancy because she needed to "focus on myself." Yet other WTS clients assumed she felt bad about having an abortion. "I feel fine," Christine declared with conviction. She was happy that she had done what was best for herself, Christine continued, saying that because she is in treatment, "I need to get other things together." Karen validated Christine's response. Focusing on the self was just what Karen and other WTS staff wanted women to do. Then, almost as an afterthought, Christine mentioned that a senior staff member had informed her that if she remained pregnant, she would be expelled from the program. Everyone in the class knew that an early discharge would look bad to the court, which had the power to send Christine to prison if she failed at WTS. Karen nodded understandingly and told the clients that while it was normal to dislike being there, rehab is one time that women can think only about themselves. Therefore, being at WTS is actually quite special. Treatment, Karen explained, "is like a spiritual retreat."

A month after Christine said that she wanted to "get other things together," she happily reported to her classmates that she had gotten a job. But the following week, Christine told me that WTS had made her quit the job. Given Americans' long-standing concern that poor people and drug users are irresponsible, I was surprised. Christine was not. Seemingly resigned, she explained that the staff felt that "I wasn't getting any treatment" because her work hours were too long. Although Christine adopted WTS's dictate to "focus on" herself, WTS got to decide what this meant. With the state's power to punish behind it, WTS made Christine give up both work and mother-hood. To become empowered, WTS insisted that women retreat from social relationships and transform themselves.

A few years later, I ventured into another residential addiction treatment program that claims to be "designed for" women. Unlike WTS, Gladstone Lodge has no relationship with the criminal justice system. Its clients are in the program voluntarily. Instead, it contracts with health insurance companies, unions, and employers. The women who enter the Lodge pay with insurance or cash just as they would for any health-care service, and as a result they are from working-class or middle-class backgrounds, and mostly white. There I witnessed different treatment methods and divergent ideas about what women need to be empowered. Treatment was not about remaking selves; it was about getting women sober.

In one session, Rayanne, a counselor, asked the clients to read a page photocopied from a book of daily thoughts and prayers inspired by the twelve steps of Alcoholics Anonymous.[2] Susan volunteered. A college-educated twenty-eight-year-old white cocaine user, Susan had admitted herself to rehab to save her relationship with her fiancé and to convince the state to reissue her driver's license, which she had lost after several arrests for driving while intoxicated. The page she read asked the women to think about how they "can live without [using] and be happy." The answer given is "fellowship" with others in Narcotics or Alcoholics Anonymous. Susan read that with sobriety, "You will know what it means to give of yourself. . . . You will become happy, respected, and useful once more." The text promised each client that she would become a "normal person" and asked all of them to pray to be "grateful" for what they have. Cathy emphatically responded that she was happy she "woke up sober today. . . . Thank God for being sober today. I like it." Alexa added that she'd always felt "useless": "I only brought pain and never brought any joy . . . I just took from the world." Sounding emotional, Alexa said she always wanted to be "normal." Through sobriety, the Lodge aimed to redeem women by return-ing them to respectability. This required them to be useful in "normal" social roles. As a result, when the program director, Ruth, heard that Susan's mother did not want her to work after treatment, she was troubled. "An addict in her own company is in very bad company," Ruth explained. Ruth resolved to convince Susan's mother that work promoted sobriety. Indeed, sobriety was so important that women were told not to make any major life changes until they had been clean for one year. Consequently, staff members discouraged white, working-class Jill from leaving her abusive husband.

WTS and Gladstone Lodge both claim to treat addiction.[3] They are licensed by the same northeastern US state to offer treatment for what is officially considered a "chronic, relapsing brain disease."[4] The people that staff both programs have similar training as licensed substance abuse counselors, and they agree on the importance of gender-sensitive rehab for women. Yet I found that WTS and Gladstone Lodge have different definitions of addiction. At the Lodge addiction meant substance abuse. There, women learned to "live sober" by "working a program" of new daily habits, renouncing selfishness, and relying on others for help. Treatment promised to make women respectable and happy "once more" by fitting them back into their lives. In contrast, WTS defined addiction as having a profoundly disordered and dependent self. This failed self led to everything from drug use to poverty to abusive relationships. At WTS, addiction was a much bigger problem, one that explained women's social marginalization. Treatment thus entailed a transformation so complete that staff members called it "habilitation," not rehabilitation. This meant "working on the self" by uncovering personal pathologies and separating from social relationships, even those with one's own children. WTS hoped this would transform "broken women" into autonomous individuals who need only themselves for fulfillment. In short, the Lodge sought to end chemical dependency, while WTS sought to end gendered dependency. As a result, women at the Lodge had to change their lifestyles, but women at WTS had to change their very selves.

These different definitions of addiction and methods of treatment have their roots in the fact that WTS and the Lodge are distinct kinds of institutions. WTS is a penal institution, and the Lodge is a health-care service. Yet both are agents of social control that seek to normalize women who are considered to be deviant. This means that both programs have to define what is wrong with their clients, determine what it means to be a normal woman and what clients need to become that way, and then develop practical techniques for shaping women.[5] I entered these programs as an ethnographer wondering how their divergent relationship to punishment would shape this process. These rehab programs govern individuals, and they are part of different systems for governing social life—systems structured by race, class, and gender inequality. What happens in the programs is shaped by these systems. I use the term "governance" to capture more than just state policy; it refers to the ideas and techniques that many institutions use to manage conduct.[6] The Lodge works primarily with private authorities like employers, families, and unions, while insurance companies and the market mediate individuals' access to the program. In contrast, WTS is part of the criminal justice system and state welfare programs. WTS and Gladstone Lodge therefore represent different modes of governing gender, ones I found were divided by race and class. The primary aims of this book are to examine how and why the programs' versions of addiction and treatment emerged, and to uncover the consequences of using addiction discourse to understand women's lives.

REHAB IS THE NEW BLACK

Addiction treatment is an increasingly important technique for managing social problems. The past four decades of war on drugs and get-tough crime policies have led to mass incarceration and its infamous racial disparities.[7] But political officials are finally challenging this punitive turn in American criminal justice. They all point to one solution: addiction treatment. For instance, in 2015 Michael Botticelli became the first director of the White House Office of National Drug Control Policy (the position commonly known as drug czar) to have a background in treatment rather than law enforcement. In a rare display of bipartisanship, the Senate unanimously approved Botticelli and the agenda he represents. During the 2015 Republican primary debates, Senator Rand Paul and Governors Chris Christie and Jeb Bush all touted mandated treatment, arguing that such treatment is more effective and just than incarceration.[8] Meanwhile, state welfare agencies, drug researchers, and advocates for women emphasize that rehab can help women escape abuse and poverty.[9] With rising concerns over opiate use, many states are scrambling to expand treatment. Even the health-care system is feeling pressure to support rehab: the Affordable Care Act, health-care reform legislation passed during the administration of President Barack Obama, requires health insurance to cover substance abuse treatment.

The idea of addiction is also a major metaphor of our time, used to understand anything deemed to be excessive or self-injurious, including caring for other people, eating sugar, or receiving government benefits.[10] We need only look to popular culture to see the concept's reach. Each year 2 percent of the US population attends an addiction self-help group like Narcotics or Alcoholics Anonymous, and recovery discourse inspired by these groups has spawned much of the enormously profitable world of self-help publishing, which has boomed since the 1970s and shapes the lives of many more Americans.[11] Addiction especially thrives in reality television. Shows like *Intervention* feature heroic counselors who help families convince their loved ones to check into posh treatment programs. On *Celebrity Rehab* and *Sex Rehab with Dr. Drew,* washed-up stars and D-list celebrities undergo treatment to rekindle their fame. *My Strange Addiction* portrays people supposedly addicted to such behaviors as eating glass, drinking human blood, and getting breast implants. More than just titillation, these shows reflect addiction's legitimacy as a way of understanding deviance. The public's interest seems especially intense and prurient in the case of women who use drugs. Throughout the 1980s and 1990s political discourse framed poor drug-using women, especially those who are African American, as monstrous so-called crack mothers and welfare queens.[12] But things play out differently for more privileged women. When the media eagerly report on the drug-addled escapades and rehab stints of celebrities like Lindsay Lohan and Amy Winehouse, the coverage lacks such damning stigma. I saw the impact of this status distinction during the spring of 2009 when one young white woman arrived at Gladstone Lodge wearing a tight T-shirt that declared, "Rehab Is the New Black."

Despite this enthusiasm for addiction treatment, we know so little about what actually happens in rehab that scholars have called it a "black box."[13] While there are a few ethnographic studies of penal rehabs, there are no studies about what happens in programs that operate outside of criminal justice or welfare systems. Even a prominent addiction scientist admitted that he knew little about daily life in such programs.[14] This book looks inside the black box to examine how programs interpret addiction, what practices they use to manage it, and how this process is gendered and racialized. The meaning of addiction is not self-evident. It has been constructed differently over time, for various social groups, and across institutions.[15] Although some scientists and government agencies have recently pushed to define addiction as a biochemical brain disorder, it is people who work in rehabs like WTS and Gladstone Lodge who construct addiction through everyday interactions in specific social contexts. These definitions are what actually matter in treatment. Yet most scholarly studies of treatment take the meaning of addiction for granted. They rely on quantitative data to measure rates of program completion, relapse, and commission of a new offense. Critics of the rehab industry's high failure rates and meager scientific grounding also assume the definition of addiction.[16] This book takes a different approach. While questions of program efficacy are important, survey data cannot reveal how counselors and clients construct addiction and recovery or why particular treatment practices emerge.

Scholars have often understood the success of the addiction framework as an example of medicalization, whereby forms of deviance—initially seen as moral or criminal problems—are transformed into medical problems handled by doctors and psychologists.[17] Disease language is indeed ubiquitous in the recovery field, but addiction is only slightly medicalized. Although substance use disorders are official psychiatric diagnoses, medical doctors play a minor role in their treatment. Instead, addiction is most often handled in self-help groups and by state-licensed counselors, whose certification typically does not require a college degree. The disease concept operates more as a way to garner legitimacy for treatment than as a technical diagnosis. Neither medicalization nor the pervasiveness of therapeutic culture can explain the differences between WTS and Gladstone Lodge. I found that rehabs and the agencies that fund them use addiction to understand and manage a wide array of problems, including poverty, crime, gender violence, and family relationships. Thus, studies of efficacy miss the complex role that rehab plays in contemporary society. The question becomes what work various authorities expect the category of addiction to do and why. Through an ethnographic comparison of a penal rehab to one with no state funding, I examine how larger patterns of governance, punishment, and inequality shape the construction of addiction and treatment techniques. How do they determine what problems fall under the aegis of addiction treatment? Why are some desires and relationships positioned as disordered and others as normal? What do the programs think are women's specific needs? How do these agencies develop therapeutic techniques? What do they see as a successful recovery? These questions hinge on the social role of punishment and how gender and race shape the way we interpret dependency.

GOVERNING THROUGH ADDICTION AND THE PUNITIVE TURN

Debates over drug policy typically hinge on whether substance abuse should be dealt with as a medical or a criminal problem. In fact, critics of mass incarceration regularly use the argument that addiction is a disease to challenge the criminal justice system's legitimate authority over drug problems. Like WTS, they think that rehab can replace punishment and avoid its racism. Similarly, some journalists have argued that the only reason we now see support for treating addicts is because the majority of opiate users are white; in contrast, when the panic over crack cocaine focused on black people in the 1980s, the response was punishment.[18] There is no doubt that drug policy has become harsher or that this process was deeply racialized; however, it is a mistake to view medicalization and criminalization as distinct and opposing responses. Medicalized efforts to treat and reform deviants have long been part of punishment. They emerged alongside the prison and spurred the development of practices like probation and parole.[19] The inclusion of psychological and therapeutic techniques into punishment is characteristic of the period that the sociologist David Garland calls "penal modernism," a rehabilitative approach that solidified during the progressive era and dominated much of the twentieth century.[20] Aptly termed "corrections," this method is based on the idea that the criminal justice system should not only punish and deter crime but also normalize lawbreakers and provide for their welfare so that they can be reintegrated into society, lead productive lives, and participate in the duties and freedoms of citizenship. While correctional normalization often enforced racism, sexism, and class exploitation, its ideology was reintegrative.

Correctionalism developed along with the welfare state, in which the government provides a safety net and shapes social processes through programs like old age insurance, unemployment benefits, college loans, and assistance to the poor. These forms of state governance share many of the same ways of thinking about and acting on social problems, producing a mode of governance termed "penal-welfare."[21] During this era, scholars noticed similarities in the practices and ideologies of penal institutions and other agents of social regulation and control. Foucault famously showed that prisons, schools, the military, and factories used similar disciplinary techniques and forms of knowledge to create similarly docile and productive people. Likewise, the sociologist Erving Goffman demonstrated that "total institutions" like prisons, mental hospitals, and the military shared practices for remaking individual selves, although their official goals differed.[22] Research also found that psychological and therapeutic strategies for governing conduct percolated widely through society, shaping workplace management, romantic relationships, child rearing, and even how individuals managed themselves.[23] From this perspective, modern punishments were just an extreme version of the regulatory practices characteristic of many modern institutions.

Penal welfarist approaches to crime declined in the United States after the 1970s. During the 1980s and 1990s, sanctions for all offenses became harsher. Gone was the rhetoric about rehabilitating offenders and ameliorating the social causes of crime. Even as addiction discourse spread through popular culture, the criminalizing approach to drugs dominated. Heightened rhetoric about the racially coded drug crack cocaine increased the public's fear of crime and support for harsh punishments.[24] Such punitive political sentiments followed increased opposition to welfare and anxiety about changing race and gender relations.[25] It was the resulting policy changes that produced mass incarceration, with rates skyrocketing 500 percent since 1973, even though crime rates decreased after 1994.[26] By 2008, when I was starting research at Gladstone Lodge, more than 2.3 million people were behind bars (a number that stabilized around 2.2 million in 2014).[27] Less well known is that the punitive turn increased other forms of punishment, too. An additional 5 million people are under criminal justice supervision through parole, probation, or community sanctions like WTS.[28]

The consequences of mass criminalization are not borne equally. The criminal justice system disproportionately targets poor and nonwhite people, especially for drug crimes—even though studies show that whites use drugs at similar rates to nonwhites. Black people make up a particularly disproportionate percentage of the incarcerated population.[29] As a result, criminalization is now a major cause of racial inequality.[30] Crime and drugs became so heavily identified with black people that being black comes with the stigma of criminality, thus limiting opportunities for employment for all black people—even those without criminal records.[31] Penal trends are also gendered. While men make up the large majority of prisoners, women's incarceration increased at a higher rate between 1980 and 2010 (646 percent) than men's (419 percent), despite women's dramatically lower involvement in crime. Drug policy drove this gendered pattern and left black women especially overrepresented in prison and jail.[32] In 2009, when I was conducting this research, these trends were at their peak, with about 198,600 women incarcerated and another 1,125,400 being punished in the community.[33]

The national panic over so-called crack babies during the 1980s and 1990s signals how the punitive turn was simultaneously gendered and racialized. The evidence for the existence of crack babies was slim at the time, and research has shown no evidence that cocaine exposure causes a debilitating syndrome.[34] But medical doctors, politicians, and the media ran with this idea, generating a classic example of what sociologists call a moral panic.[35] Crack mothers and babies were ubiquitously depicted as black and poor. Crack was said to make women sexually voracious and to destroy "maternal instinct."[36] The rhetoric was so overheated that in 1994 the prestigious Center on Addiction and Substance Abuse at Columbia University declared pregnant women's drug use "a slaughter of innocents of biblical proportions."[37] Politicians and researchers claimed that these children would be developmentally delayed, lack morality, and become so-called super predators.[38] Drug-using African American women were especially blamed for causing poverty, crime, the decline of the traditional family, teen pregnancy, educational failure, and excessive government spending. As a result, some municipalities instituted drug testing for women in labor and newborns. Doctors reported positive tests to the police, who charged women with drug-related offences simply for being pregnant— meaning that legal action would not have been taken otherwise.[39] One study found that doctors were ten times more likely to report pregnant black women to the police for drug use than pregnant white women, even though the two groups used drugs at the same rate.[40]

Most accounts of this punitive turn argue that the criminal justice system dropped the goals of rehabilitating and normalizing individuals in favor of merely controlling and containing disadvantaged groups, particularly African Americans.[41] In short, these scholars argue that it transformed America into a penal state. This term describes a mode of state governance that relies heavily on criminalization and carceral methods to regulate the marginalized. The penal state makes extensive use of formal criminal punishment, but it also relies on a web of practices that mimic the ideologies and techniques of penal sanctions.[42] Social policy also became harsher, most famously during the 1996 welfare reform that ended poor families' entitlement to assistance and forced single mothers to work, no matter what their circumstances.[43] This shift challenges Foucault's and Goffman's emphasis on modern society's widely shared strategies of control. The sociologist Loïc Wacquant argues that we now see bifurcated governance, with punishment for the poor and nonwhite and more liberal, welfarist strategies for the privileged.[44]

The rise of the penal state has had repercussions across society. The law professor Jonathan Simon argues that crime and punishment now serve as metaphors through which many institutions understand and manage social problems, an approach he calls "governing through crime."[45] This not only expands the role of the justice system, it also opens up new sites and techniques of regulation. Simon shows that noncriminal justice institutions also govern through crime, spreading techniques such as drug testing, risk management, security cameras, and zero-tolerance policies to benefit programs, schools, workplaces, and shopping malls. Governing through crime displaced the governmental strategies characteristic of penal welfarism, such as education, moral reform, and social services.[46] For example, the welfare state overtly governs poverty through crime. Drug offenses can render individuals ineligible for federal college loans, income assistance, and public housing, thus denying them social citizenship. Notions of risk shape how this plays out along class and race lines. While marginalized populations and poor areas are seen as risky and tend to be criminalized, more privileged individuals and officials in more privileged spaces increasingly seek to manage the risk of victimization and ensure security before all else.[47] However, when parole authorities test a woman for drug use and send her to WTS or when a company tests an employee and sends her to Gladstone Lodge, crime is not the only logic at work.

I build on Simon's work to argue that we are also governing through addiction. I use this term to describe the process whereby logics and techniques from the addiction recovery field underpin how we think about and act on social relations. Many institutions govern through addiction, but this approach is most deeply rooted in punishment. It is therefore differentiated along class and race lines. The punitive turn did not eliminate efforts to reform criminalized individuals, but they do not look like they did during the heyday of penal welfarism.[48] They have been reconfigured primarily through the framework of addiction. Although addiction treatment predates the punitive turn, governing through addiction emerged as a result of governing through crime. It depends on many of the punitive and security-oriented techniques that Simon identifies. In the criminal justice system, risk management spurred the reenvisioning and expansion of rehabilitation to reduce recidivism, over-crowding, and costs.[49] As the penal system attempts to measure and address risk, it not only looks at a person's criminal history, but it also defines some individual needs, such as for housing or trauma counseling, as risks worthy of remediation because these needs correlate with recidivism. Drug abuse is prominent among the targeted risks. In the process of managing this risk, the scope, institutional form, and ideologies of contemporary punishment change.[50] Addiction treatment is therefore an important and understudied part of the penal state.

Addiction treatment has thrived because of the punitive turn, where it is used to manage the institutional crises created by mass incarceration. The sociologist Jill McCorkel found that a women's prison created a harsh drug treatment program in response to overcrowding and an increasingly black population. These changes delegitimated the prison's traditional rehabilitative orientation based on the idea that inmates were "good girls" who had been led astray by bad men. Instead, prison officials viewed the racialized inmates as "real criminals" with permanently disordered selves.[51] The treatment program offered a solution to this crisis because it enabled the prison to get tough and hold women accountable, while also seeming to be gender appropriate. Gov-erning through addiction diversifies the forms that punishment can take, often locating it in community-based programs like WTS while drawing on new ideologies. The most distinctive vehicle for this change has been drug courts, where people like Christine are sentenced to rehab and intensively monitored by the court according to therapeutic standards that merge recovery discourse with legal notions of accountability.

As a result of these processes, the penal state is particularly entwined with treatment. Criminal justice institutions are the largest single source of referrals to rehab, accounting for 37 percent of the over 1.8 million admis-sions to treatment in 2010.[52] State funding for rehab has exploded since 1997, when the federal government started collecting data. Back then, only 16.1 percent of rehab facilities received federal, state, or local funding, but by 2010, 61.6 percent of them did.[53] Public monies accounted for 69 percent of all substance abuse treatment spending in 2009, while private insurance paid for only 16 percent.[54] When I began my research at WTS in 2004, I was unaware of how foundational addiction discourse was to its approach. Since then, nearly all ethnographic studies of penal treatment and reentry programs have found that they focus on addiction or rely on ideas and techniques from the recovery field, even when addressing seemingly unre-lated issues like job readiness.[55] Other parts of the penal state use similar techniques to manage marginalized populations, such as when recipients of public assistance are screened and tested for drug use.[56] In many states, individuals can regain eligibility for welfare only by going to rehab.[57] Teresa Gowan's research revealed that the main way homeless men could get off the street was to enter rehab—that was the approach that all services were taking.[58] Even the police have gotten on board. Forrest Stuart found that Los Angeles Police Department officers in Skid Row push the homeless into treatment programs and view their role as "recovery managers."[59] Governing through addiction thereby links punishment and welfare through agencies like WTS.

The gender politics of the punitive turn shape how governing through addiction operates. Although men are the majority of people in rehab, women are especially likely to have their problems viewed through the lens of addiction. Since correctional officials tend to consider women to be at lower risk of committing violence and more psychologically troubled than men, they are preferred candidates for diversion into treatment. Moreover, women's experiences of gender violence, child care, and romantic relationships are constructed as risks that require penal treatment.[60] Notions of personal disorder and illness fit with stereotypes about women and echo older penal welfarist approaches that normalized women into traditional feminine roles. Yet as McCorkel's research shows, racist and sexist tropes from the punitive turn make addiction an especially appealing logic in contemporary punishment.[61] Nevertheless, addiction discourse is not always associated with gender traditionalism. Theorists of "gender-responsive" treatment, which is influential in the criminal justice system, argue that it can actually challenge women's subordination and the sexist racism that fostered mass incarceration.[62]

Scholars of penal rehab are less sanguine. They argue it extends the state's power to punish in part because it is premised on addiction ideology. Drug courts, for instance, frame users as permanently sick and therefore permanently bad. Thus punishment, including incarceration, becomes the treatment.[63] The sociologist Lynne Haney researched a community-based prison for mothers and children that was organized, like my sites, around gender-sensitive treatment. Instead of education or job training, the treatment included spa days and yoga, but its centerpiece was harrowing, confrontational group therapy that forced women to repeatedly recount painful experiences like rape in the name of healing the self. These practices left women devastated and damaged their relationships with their children. The prison rehab that McCorkel studied also made women undergo humiliating therapy "with the goal of breaking down" their "diseased selves."[64] It was so brutal that some participants even asked to be transferred back to regular prison. This method stemmed from a belief that the prisoners would forever be addicts and must surrender to a treatment process, which, like at WTS, was called habilitation. McCorkel argues that habilitation indicates the abandonment of rehabilitation, replacing it with the continual penal supervision of marginalized groups.

Governing through addiction also occurs in institutional arenas outside the penal state. Private authorities' use of rehab has partly been driven by state policy, such as the Drug Free Workplaces Act of 1988 that required that federal contractors and grantees maintain drug-free workplaces. Insurance companies began to cover chemical dependency in the 1970s and thereby expanded rehab.[65] Meanwhile, scientists, self-help publishers, and advocates of twelve-step programs operated as moral entrepreneurs, promoting the idea that addiction was a key social problem and legitimating the notion that recovery from it would address various social ills.[66] Their message was aligned with broader cultural and structural changes that made emotional fulfillment a central life goal and rendered individuals responsible for cultivating themselves to achieve success in economic and personal matters.[67] As a result, individuals also govern themselves through addiction when they apply recovery discourse to their lives. Together, these forces rendered addiction an appealing and useful framework for interpreting and managing social, relational, and individual problems. Although private authorities and health-care institutions are lesser players in the rehab system as a whole, the push to expand access to treatment will enlarge their role and increase the number of middle-class people in the system. The spread of governing through addiction raises questions about whether and how penal institutions share ideologies and techniques with other forms of social control and, more broadly, what this tells us about the nature of contemporary governance.

WTS and Gladstone Lodge share many classic disciplinary techniques and draw on similar discourses. They take people away from everyday life to live collectively, following similar schedules, within a more or less closed institutional environment. Like the total institutions Goffman studied, these rehabs label their clients and try to get women to see themselves through this new identity. In keeping with Foucault's famous argument, both facilities subject women to surveillance to gather information to diagnose and control them. Women spend most of their time doing group therapy and completing written exercises in which they must confess their failings and learn new ways of managing their own conduct. Both WTS and the Lodge also work within the recovery culture. Not only were their staff members trained in it, but many counselors were also recovering addicts. Consequently, even staff members of the Lodge would share some of the assumptions made by staffers at the harsh prison rehab that McCorkel studied: addiction is a permanent disease that requires addicts to surrender to treatment. Most notably, both WTS and the Lodge used addiction discourse to understand gender. Their staff members argued that women with addiction suffer from trauma, codependency, and low self-esteem. They believed that men often introduce women to using, and that men's violence against women fuels addiction. I can easily imagine counselors from both programs getting along famously as they chatted about how the world judges women who use drugs more harshly than male users and commiserated about how women don't get treatment because they are expected to sacrifice themselves for children and men. The counselors would agree that in rehab, women should focus on themselves.

Nevertheless, these shared ideas and techniques did not translate into similar constructions of addiction or methods of treatment. Gladstone Lodge's definition of "addiction" was narrow, and the program's treatment focused on changing women's lifestyle so they could be reintegrated into society and reclaim their status as respectable. Although the Lodge depended on forms of coercion, labeled women with the deviant identity of addict, and attempted to normalize them into conventional roles, it had much less power over them than WTS had over its clients. Women at the Lodge were customers, from higher class backgrounds, and were not criminalized. In contrast, WTS was fundamentally more punitive. The threat of prison backed the program's power, and this showed in its therapeutic and disciplinary methods. By keeping women from motherhood, employment, and personal life, WTS suspended women's citizenship just like a more traditional punishment.[68] Moreover, its notion of addiction invoked tropes of criminality. I argue that this difference reveals the hallmarks of punishment: its distinctive ability to stigmatize and coerce. It is these features that distinguish punishment, even in therapeutic guise, from other forms of social control. I draw on theories of punishment that suggest punishment is not just about controlling people (although it surely does that). It also has a unique ability to create meaning by marking individuals as degraded others. Punishment thereby produces and reproduces social boundaries.[69] In the current moment, this means that penal rehab programs not only define addiction, but they are also "race-making."[70] WTS constructed a distinctive type of addiction premised on the racialized and gendered stigmas associated with the punitive turn, while the Lodge worked hard to dissociate its clients from such disreputable addicts. This stigma turns on the politics of dependency.

GENDER, RACE, AND THE POLITICS OF DEPENDENCY

Feminist scholars have examined how systems of state regulation are organized around particular symbols or "signs," often deeply resonant constructions of what is masculine and feminine.[71] These symbols shape how state welfare regimes are structured; the techniques of regulation they use; and the relationships they create among individuals, families, workplaces, markets, and the state.[72] For example, the idea of the dependent mother and her opposition to the masculine, independent, paid worker shaped the US welfare state into two gendered wings. In one wing, workers (coded as male) are rights-bearing individuals who are entitled to social insurance programs like Social Security. In the other, mothers are dependents who participate in the stigmatized, need-based assistance program we typically think of as welfare, where they are subjected to surveillance and normalization. The meaning of these signs can change, as was the case in the 1996 welfare reform that created the program Temporary Assistance to Needy Families (TANF). Nancy Fraser and Linda Gordon argue that before then, women's dependence had been seen as natural, while men's was deviant.[73] But through discourses about so-called welfare queens, poor women were racialized as black and stigmatized as pathologically dependent. To cure this, welfare reform claimed to promote independence by making women work for pay rather than in the home. In the process of allocating rights and defining needs through tropes of dependence and independence, these signs constructed gendered forms of citizenship. In the current context, addiction is just such a sign.

Governing through addiction is reconfiguring the relationship between punishment and welfare provision, especially for women. The rhetoric of the punitive turn fueled this process. In response to the crack baby panic, the federal government expanded funding for gender-specialized addiction treatment even as local prosecutors were criminalizing women.[74] At the same time, child welfare agencies adopted zero-tolerance policies toward parental drug use, treating it more seriously than child abuse or neglect. These cases are disproportionately brought against women, especially women of color.[75] Child welfare agencies send the women in such cases to treatment. Addiction acts as a framing device for the social safety net—one that is typically delivered through criminalization. Indeed, advocates of drug courts gush that they are a "unique service delivery system."[76] Consequently, women can get many more services at WTS than in any other government program. This is because it receives funding not only from parole and drug courts, but also from the city's child protective services (CPS) agency, programs that combat homelessness, and TANF. Places like WTS therefore coordinate the penal system and welfare state through the idea of addiction. Women end up at WTS not only because they are criminalized, but also because they are poor. The pathways women in my study took to WTS were therefore different than the ones women took to Gladstone Lodge. People with means or jobs with benefits can use insurance or their own funds to pay for rehab. While the Lodge participates in this work-based system for providing social goods, WTS operates in a different circuit designed for poor women. These inequalities stratify treatment, resulting in modes of governance that are bifurcated by race and class. I argue that within the penal system, governing through addiction is a strategy for managing social marginalization. This new configuration of penal welfare rests on differently gendered constructions of dependency than did welfare reform.

Fraser and Gordon reveal that construction of the welfare queen was distinctive because her dependency is not just financial—it is also psychological. Sanford Schram argues that this notion of pathological dependency is credited with shifting welfare "from an income redistribution scheme to a behavior modification scheme."[77] What is less well known is that this version of dependency derives from addiction recovery discourse about women. When WTS staffers claimed that women "didn't even have a self" yet and when they worried about women's desire to mother their children or have romantic relationships, they were diagnosing women with codependency. This concept derives from twelve-step culture and describes a person's overreliance on external sources of meaning and validation that manifests itself in her desire to care for others and in substance abuse. Codependency is stereotypically associated with women. The gender studies scholar Trysh Travis argues that it operates as a critique of women's position in the family and their traditional obligation to sacrifice themselves to care for men and children.[78] However, codependency also suggests that women's selves are the source of these inequities. This concept is widespread in the recovery field. At both WTS and Gladstone Lodge, it served as the primary way to understand gender oppression. Like WTS staffers, Lodge counselors also worried about women's codependent relationships and the burdens of care work. Yet because its clients were seen as respectable and the Lodge was beholden to their families and employers, staff members there did not try to modify women's relationships or change the gendered aspects of their selves—even with black clients. This would be stigmatizing. Instead, the Lodge emphasized using the twelve steps and help from other women to stay sober so clients could resume these very roles. This was not what happened at WTS.

Codependency discourse has been framed as a very middle-class trend,[79] but it is thriving at WTS and in other penal institutions. However, governing through addiction looks different for men. They are not dependent. Miranda March's research at a program much like WTS revealed that its staff members diagnosed women as suffering from dependence and low self-esteem. Meanwhile at a men's program just a few blocks away, staff members saw clients as rational actors who willfully chose the pleasures of the street over productive, masculine work. Similarly, in a study of how probation and parole officers view their clients, Jessica Wyse discovered that although they believed men to be irresponsible and immature, they considered women to have weak selves and to be unable to control their emotions and function independently of others.[80] At WTS, codependency defined addiction, making gender deviance the cause of women's problems. The program therefore targeted the gendered aspects of women's selves—everything from mothering and clothing choices to rape trauma. As my analysis will show, in the context of punishment, code-pendency and addiction become deeply racialized because they fit with char-acterizations of the welfare queen and cultural explanations of poverty. This enabled WTS to pathologize women's motherhood and families. Even more than prior welfare regimes, governing through addiction turns social inequal-ity into women's psychological problems.

THE RESEARCHER GOES TO REHAB:
RESEARCH METHODS AND SITE SELECTION

The research for this comparative ethnography was conducted in two phases, one at WTS in 2004–5 and the other at Gladstone Lodge in 2008–9. At each site, I spent about seven months regularly observing the program, visiting about two times a week. I did fieldwork at both sites less often for another three to four months. I collected data at the two sites a few years apart because I did not originally intend to do a comparative study. What I found at WTS raised theoretical and empirical questions that required comparative analysis. I began my research at WTS wondering whether and how the racial-ized politics about drug-using women shaped the way the program under-stood and regulated women, particularly regarding mothering. I was surprised at the staff's emphasis on women's self-esteem and pathological dependence on children. That did not fit with what we knew about gendered governance, which suggested that the welfare state disciplined poor women into low-wage labor, while rhetoric about drug-using mothers damned them for violating traditional norms of motherhood. What is more, other sociologists soon found similar patterns in women's penal institutions. Something was going on. I realized that what connects these criminal justice institutions is their use of an addiction framework. This raised theoretical questions about the nature of punishment, the role of addiction discourse, and how race and class intersect with gender in institutions whose aim is to normalize and control women. I needed to study an addiction rehab that was outside the penal state but oth-erwise similar. To find a comparison site I looked for all-women rehabs that had no relationship with the criminal justice system and accepted no public funding. This led me to Gladstone Lodge.

WTS and the Lodge are not representative in the statistical sense (indeed, being women-only makes them unusual); however, they are well suited to this comparison.[81] My goal was to ethnographically examine how larger processes of governance and inequality impinge on the micro level of treatment. These two programs are as ideal case studies as is possible given the structural differ-ences between the penal and private-pay systems of addiction treatment. This is because they differ in a theoretically and empirically revealing way—their relationship to the penal state—while also sharing many key characteristics. They are located in the same northeastern state and regulated by the same state agency. They also share the stated goal of providing gender-sensitive treatment. Both are residential and abstinence-based; however, women at the Lodge have much shorter treatment times due to insurance constraints. WTS offers more services and a softer approach than most penal rehabs. This distinctiveness is actually a virtue: it means that WTS is a best-case scenario of what treatment advocates want. As a sex-segregated program, the Lodge is among the minority of private-pay rehabs. However, it is typical in one significant way: it follows the classic twelve-step model that dominates the field (especially in private-paid programs). Given the racial patterns in criminal justice and jobs with benefits, I was not surprised to find that the client population at the Lodge was whiter and wealthier than that at WTS. But because of the Lodge's relationship to unions, its clients are not especially privileged: they are working-class and middle-class women. The Lodge is therefore a modest, low-cost inpatient rehab—not the sort of place where celebrities go.

My data are drawn primarily from my ethnographic observations, supplemented with two other sources: program documents and my interviews with staff members. In addition to many informal conversations with staff members and clients during everyday life, I conducted open-ended interviews with key staffers. Finally, I collected and analyzed therapeutic texts and administrative documents from each program. These included worksheets, readings, intake forms, promotional materials, treatment planning tools, and case reports. During my ethnographic fieldwork, I sat in on staff meetings, group-therapy sessions (referred to simply as "group"), and special events. I hung out during meals and breaks with both staff members and clients. Because I was interested in the institutions' culture, mode of therapeutic governance, and relationship to larger systems, I spent more time with staff members than I did with clients. To avoid making people uncomfortable or changing the social dynamics, I did not usually take notes during therapeutic groups.[82] I jotted down field notes during breaks and in some meetings. I then took detailed field notes after leaving the site.

On the whole, I had more access at Gladstone Lodge than at WTS. This was for three reasons. First, the Lodge has a smaller number of both clients and staff members, and they have almost the same schedule every day. Thus, I could observe most facets of the program and meet everyone. In contrast, WTS is larger and busier, and it has a complex schedule. Several groups run simultaneously, and clients regularly come and go to work and appointments or leave early. This made it hard for me to meet all the clients and to pin down staffers to talk. Second, I was able to stay overnight at the Lodge several times because it had the room. This enabled me to spend more time with clients while they were not in group sessions than I could at WTS. Third, as a white woman I was more of an outsider at WTS because the majority of its staff members and clients were black or Latina. It is surely the case that my race and class status distanced me from some people at WTS, while it facilitated my relationship with people at the Lodge. Although I cannot know what individuals really thought of me, I believe that I gained a rapport with some WTS women, and many WTS clients shared their criticisms of the program with me. Yet in some ways, I fit in more easily at WTS, which had interns and volunteers, than I did in the Lodge's familial culture.

OVERVIEW

My ethnographic analysis begins by situating both programs in their respective institutional arenas. Chapter 1 describes WTS and Gladstone Lodge in detail and analyzes the structure of governing through addiction. I reveal that treatment is a two-tiered system, divided by race and class. By tracing the pathways women take to rehab, I show how each site is linked to distinct systems of governance. These pathways reflect the history of how state policy, gender ideology, and social stratification have shaped addiction treatment since its earliest days. These larger patterns shape why, how, and where people go to treatment, leading to race and class differences in the programs' client populations. Moreover, they shape the power each rehab has over women. Although funders and referral agencies all govern through addiction, I argue that these systems produce different treatment structures and services. Paradoxically, these forces make WTS much more generous than the Lodge, but they do not mean that WTS women have worse drug problems than those at the Lodge. The clients at both programs have many needs, so staff members must do interpretive work to determine which are their responsibilities and how to address them.

My ethnographic analysis of WTS takes place in chapters 2 and 3. In chapter 2, I unpack WTS's definition of addiction and show how this was related to its role in the criminal justice system. WTS staff members spent surprisingly little time worrying about women's drug use or criminal behavior. Instead, addiction meant having a weak, dependent self. Clients' experiences with drugs, crime, prostitution, and abusive boyfriends were merely symptoms of their "addiction to pain and punishment." Habilitation therefore targets the self, not a woman's social situation. I argue that this version of addiction reflects the racial and gender politics of contemporary punishment. This chapter shows how WTS remained punitive not despite but because of its addiction framework. Criminal punishment, I argue, entails a unique power to control and stigmatize. At WTS, this stigma is profoundly racialized. WTS ultimately marks racial, gender, and class boundaries, and it unwittingly joins the prison in furthering the marginalization of poor women. Chapter 3 describes what the process of habilitation entailed, examining why women had to reform the gendered aspects of their lives and why they were often prevented from mothering their children. WTS staff members were right to worry about women's ability to meet normative standards. Most women struggle to have it all, and WTS's marginalized clients had to survive in a world where they could, in fact, expect little from the state or the labor market. The program could do nothing to change this, so the staff opted for training women to need as little as possible from other people or society. Women had to disengage from social ties in order to fix their selves by delving into their trauma and emotions and undergoing makeovers. The WTS staff thought that this process empowered women. Drawing on theories of intersectionality, I reveal how reforming gender was also a way of reforming class and race.

In chapters 4 and 5, I turn to Gladstone Lodge. There, addiction meant chemical dependency. Because of this different notion of dependency, treatment did not require a wholesale transformation of the self. It required getting sober by diligently "working" the twelve steps. The Lodge defined addiction this way because of how it constructed the clients and the program itself. Avoiding criminal justice funding was a way to get what staffers considered to be morally superior addicts, ones who they claimed were respectable "working people" like them. They contrasted their clients with the criminalized ones in rehabs like WTS, whom they racialized as "off the street" and in need of "habilitation." With the expansion of penal rehab and the declining security of the working-class people the Lodge serves, staffers felt the program and their social respectability were under threat. Thus, treatment at the Lodge promised redemption not from the addict label itself, but from its racial, class, and gender stigma. Chapter 5 brings gender into my intersectional analysis of the Lodge's methods. Counselors were aware of the gendered constraints clients faced and often criticized the sexism they encountered at work, but the program did not view gendered deviance as the cause of addiction. Limited by stingy health insurance funding and committed to the belief in their clients' essential respectability, the Lodge's counselors taught a new sober lifestyle. To do this, staff members battled what they considered to be women's selfishness. A key goal was to convince women that they could not rely solely on themselves. This also meant that they were not responsible for everything in their lives and deserved help. Consequently, the program focused on reintegrating women into social life, through bonding with other women addicts and strengthening ties with family and work.

In the conclusion of the book, I consider what this comparison tells us about governing through addiction, punishment, and the social control of gender. Ideas about dependence and independence are central to defining not just addiction but also citizenship, autonomy, and equality. Thus WTS and the Lodge had to navigate competing ideals about women's role in society, especially regarding mothering, work, and relationships. In short, they had to wrestle with the value of individualism and the nature of women's subordination. The counselors at both programs were not gender conservatives. They cared for the women they treated. But by using addiction frameworks to understand and respond to these problems, they individualized women's subordination and rendered them responsible for managing it. Ultimately WTS and Gladstone Lodge came to different conclusions about what women need to live equal and fulfilled lives. According to the Lodge, women needed and deserved help, and they deserved to be part of society. But according to WTS, the criminalized women there had to learn to live without social support and to need only themselves. The spread of governing women through addiction suggests the emergence of a new framework for understanding gender. That framework not only fails to tackle gender inequality, it also reproduces racial and class marginalization.

CHAPTER 1

Intake

PATHWAYS TO TREATMENT

SARAH ENDED UP IN REHAB because of a doctor. A white woman in her late thirties, Sarah works as a nurse; she also wrote herself illegal prescriptions for the oxycodone-containing drug Percocet by using the name of a doctor who was both a colleague and a friend. Sarah funded her habit by stealing thousands of dollars from her father while managing his finances. Despite efforts to control the misuse of prescription opiates, it was a while before Sarah got caught. Finally, a suspicious pharmacist called the doctor whose name was on the prescriptions. Although he was unaware of Sarah's actions, he covered for her to prevent her from losing her nursing license. He also called her husband. Together with her children, they lured Sarah home with a story about how her daughter had been injured and staged an intervention. The doctor promised not to report Sarah if she got help, and he recommended she go to Gladstone Lodge because that was where his own daughter had gone for treatment. After an arduous withdrawal in a detox clinic, Sarah was lucky to spend four weeks at the Lodge—the longest stretch of inpatient treatment that her insurance would cover. Sarah felt awful about what she had done, but she found solace at the Lodge, where she met four other nurses. Finding people in the same boat made her "feel like a person" and reassured her that she was "not so bad."

Donisha also had a brush with medical authorities before coming to rehab, but hers was a more formal and coercive route. About the same age as Sarah, Donisha is a black woman whose pathway to rehab started after she gave birth and tested positive for an illegal drug. The hospital reported her to the city's child protective services (CPS) agency, which placed her baby daughter in foster care. The family court overseeing the case required Donisha to complete one year of residential treatment at Women's Treatment Services (WTS). This made her one of only three WTS clients who did not have a criminal justice mandate to be in the program. Donisha proudly described herself to me as a "voluntary" client, distinguishing herself from those with a "criminal" label. Indeed, she was technically voluntary. Yet Donisha was similar to her peers. She had been in prison before, long enough that the state had terminated her parental rights to two children, a situation that is common among incarcerated women.[1] Moreover, if Donisha did not successfully graduate from WTS, she would lose custody of her new baby. While at WTS, she was eager to get a general equivalency diploma (GED) and job training and to be reunited with her daughter. However, these priorities came into conflict with those of WTS. Donisha said that the staff made her feel like a "fuck-up" and asked her to degrade herself. Eventually, she left the program without permission, which the criminal justice system terms "absconding."

Although Sarah and Donisha both used drugs and broke the law, they took different pathways to rehab, ended up in different kinds of programs, and thus had different experiences in treatment. Charting what I call pathways to treatment reveals a great deal about WTS, Gladstone Lodge, and how we govern through addiction. In this chapter, I trace the processes by which women enter these two rehabs. The pathways concept captures the social relationships and institutions that push women to seek treatment, shape what kind of program they go to, and fund treatment. They are, in short, pathways for people, money, and power. Underpinning these pathways are larger systems of inequality and governance, such as patterns in employment, workplace benefits, criminal justice processes, the welfare state, and informal familial relationships.

I suspected that the women at the Lodge would be more privileged than those at WTS, but I was unsure how much the treatment practices would differ. What I found were two nearly distinct systems of treatment and client populations. Yet in interviews of staff members at WTS or the Lodge, I found that they often used the same language to discuss addiction and women's needs. Concealed under this ubiquitous recovery lingo are two kinds of rehab programs whose different structures, services, and populations hint at their distinct social roles. This distinction may appear to be one of medicalization versus criminalization. However, neither program was especially medicalized. Moreover, the treatment system funnels people into rehab based not on a diagnosis of the nature or severity of their substance use, but rather on their socioeconomic status and relationship to the penal state. As a result, the pathways women take to Gladstone Lodge and WTS reveal addiction treatment to be a two-tiered system embedded in structures of racial, class, and gender inequality. These intersecting axes of inequality position people differently within systems of governance, sending them along different pathways.

MEDICALIZATION, CRIMINALIZATION, AND THE HISTORY OF ADDICTION TREATMENT

For WTS and Gladstone Lodge, it all started in the 1970s with nuns. Nuns founded WTS in a northeastern US city to serve as a halfway house for women leaving prison. It was not originally an addiction treatment program. In keeping with penal-welfarist ideas about rehabilitation, the nuns focused on teaching women blue-collar trades, but rather unusually these included traditionally male-dominated fields. Today, WTS is a nonprofit organization that has no religious affiliation—although a statue of the Virgin Mary still sits by the front door. Instead, it survived by formalizing its relationship with the state and tapping into the criminal justice system's deep pockets. As ideas about why women commit crimes shifted away from social and moral explanations,[2] WTS's approach to rehabilitation also changed. The program no longer emphasizes reintegrating former prisoners into society through work or religion. Now, addiction provides the framework for understanding women's deviance.

Located about a two-hour drive away from WTS, Gladstone Lodge is a for-profit, residential treatment facility that was founded in the 1970s by Bill and Faye, an older white couple who still own and run the program. They are recovering alcoholics who got sober in Alcoholics Anonymous (AA), and they remain deeply devoted to the twelve-step model of treatment. Both Catholic, Faye and Bill opened the Lodge on the grounds of a convent, in a building that had once housed tuberculosis patients. The nuns provided the only affordable space for the couple's precariously funded business. While the Lodge is no longer in that location, statues of the Virgin Mary and other saints stand by the front door, echoing the entrance to WTS. This similarity was an unplanned and surprising coincidence in my research. However, the programs' shared roots in religious outreach and their trajectories since then hint at how governing through addiction has expanded and at how the treatment field bifurcated as it became integrated with the penal state.

The 1970s were a moment of growth for addiction treatment programs. This was the era when the contemporary system of specialized addiction rehab programs took shape. Two factors contributed to this expansion. The first was an influx of government funding for addiction treatment; the second was that health insurers began to consider alcoholism an insurable illness.[3] These two relationships—to state agendas (especially about the marginalized) and the private health-care system—have structured the treatment system since the earliest institutions devoted to treating addiction, the inebriate asylums of the late nineteenth century.[4] Moreover the ambivalence of both the state and medicine has kept the addiction recovery field decentralized, semiprofessionalized, and estranged from mainstream health care. Since the days of inebriate asylums, this dynamic has reflected the shifting racial, class, and gender stigmas around substance use.

The nineteenth-century idea of inebriety marks the first effort to medicalize this problem and develop professional treatment. The notion that chronic substance abuse is a disease—meaning that people imbibe not because they want to but because they are compelled to do so—dates from around 1800, and it began in the days when early temperance advocates made alcohol the first problem drug. Before the mid-nineteenth century, Americans problematized drunkenness as a willful sin.[5] For people with property, drunkenness itself was not a problem. Poor drunkards, however, were a problem because they could not support themselves. They were lumped in with paupers, orphans, and other groups considered to be dependent. Early Americans did not distinguish between being poor and being deviant—a merging that continues in some contemporary penal rehabs.[6] Thus, poor drunkards fell under the purview of the newly emerging carceral institutions for managing poverty and deviance: prisons, workhouses, and lunatic asylums. But these institutions did not want drunkards or their moral stigma.[7] Meanwhile, narcotics use was common in the nineteenth century, especially among middle-class women who, like Sarah, took opiates as medicine. However, women alcoholics received extra stigma for violating gender norms, and many were imprisoned for inebriety.[8]

Criminal and gendered stigmas continue to shape the construction of addiction and the treatment field, ultimately spurring its bifurcation along lines of class and race. Early temperance advocates pressed for voluntary pledges of abstinence, but as drinking became associated with immigrants and the urban poor in the late nineteenth century, the advocates' approach shifted toward criminalization.[9] At the same time, some members of the newly solidified medical profession attempted to claim ownership of this problem. They expanded the category of inebriety to include other drugs but applied it only to users who were white and well-to-do.[10] The drunken poor and Chinese opium smokers remained sinners. Because the disease concept allowed drug and alcohol users to remain members of the moral community, early treatment programs were not a way of dealing with people who were considered to be social others. Consequently, most of the people in inebriate asylums were affluent men.[11] At the time, treatment included everything from whole-grain cereal to cocaine.[12] However, "moral treatment" was the dominant method and laid the foundation for rehab today. It involved removing patients from their environment to "well-ordered," family-like institutions where they prepared to reenter middle-class life through learning self-control, praying, and engaging in productive work.[13]

Inebriate asylums disappeared rapidly after 1900. William White, a historian of addiction treatment, argues that their competition with temperance's moral model and inebriety's contested status within medicine left these institutions poorly integrated into the emerging penal welfare system, which supported the development of insane asylums and reformatories.[14] In contrast to these organizations, inebriate asylums often failed to secure state funding or the backing of involuntary commitment laws. Early addiction treatments, therefore, operated on the outskirts of medicine with close ties to religious revivals, popular movements, and shady businessmen. Inebriate treatment fully collapsed after passage of the 1914 Harrison Narcotics Tax Act and Prohibition in 1919, when the problem moved decidedly into the realm of crime.[15] Mariana Valverde argues that addiction remains quasi-medicalized because of this moral stigma, producing the low-status, stratified, and paraprofessional system of today.[16]

The end of inebriate asylums left few formal treatment options, a situation that persisted until the 1960s. People could go to a psychiatric hospital or buy supposed cures (usually full of alcohol) sporting names such as Howe's Arabian Tonic and Mensman's Peptonized Beef Tonic.[17] With the criminalization of doctor-supplied opiate maintenance, the archetypal drug addict shifted from an ailing, middle-class white woman to a nonwhite, urban man who was orientalized as effeminate. This cemented the association of narcotics with racial minorities and gendered deviance.[18] Criminalization did not eliminate treatment. The one treatment organization that expanded in the early twentieth century was the penal institution called an inebriate farm, where poor people spent their days in hard labor and faced sterilization under eugenics laws.[19] There were few treatments for illegal drug users until the federal government created two penal institutions known as narcotics farms to alleviate prison overcrowding. The farms lasted into the 1970s but sought to exclude women altogether or limit their numbers. Because there are fewer of them, the added stigma of their gender, and their poor fit with male-dominated models of addiction, women are marginalized and underserved in the treatment field to this day.[20]

Into this treatment gap stepped AA. Founded in 1935, this group would forever change the construction of addiction and its treatment. AA began with two middle-class white men who had failed at numerous medical and religious cures for alcoholism. Drawing on Protestant self-help practices, AA bucked the authority of medical professionals and emphasized the power of groups of alcoholics—mostly white men in the early days—who came together to support each other's sobriety. AA used the language of disease to account for why members felt unable to control their drinking when other people could. AA also sought to reassure outsiders that they were not morally prudish prohibitionists akin to members of the temperance movement. The goal of the disease language was to show that AA members did not blame alcohol. Instead, they blamed themselves.[21] Given its deprofessionalized origins, AA's success is nothing short of astonishing. It played a key role in promoting the disease concept and spurred the creation of private alcoholism rehabs in the 1950s, and its theories continue to influence scientific models of addiction.[22]

Neither Sarah nor Donisha would have ended up in rehab without the idea that addiction is a disease, but medicine played a small role in their treatment. The success of AA's barely medicalized disease concept garnered state support for rehab outside medicine, including within penal institutions. In 1966, the Narcotic Addict Rehabilitation Act, a federal civil commitment law that permitted states to coerce individuals into rehab, created community-based treatment programs and opened the door for people other than physicians to treat addiction. In 1970, just before the punitive turn, the Comprehensive Alcohol Abuse and Alcoholism Prevention, Treatment, and Rehabilitation Act (referred to as the Hughes Act) poured more money into alcoholism treatment and research. Although drug and alcohol treatment remained separate until the 1980s, these two laws created the system we have today. Constance Weisner and Robin Room argue that this funding boom expanded the category of addiction and made treatment more coercive.[23] In fact, by 1974, Senator Harold Hughes, who introduced the 1970 act, seemed disturbed by what he had created, calling it the "alcohol and drug industrial complex."[24] When funding and insurance coverage were expanded, it was members of twelve-step programs like Faye and Bill who were there to use it. As a result, nearly all contemporary rehabs still rely on twelve-step ideology and techniques.[25]

GLADSTONE LODGE AND THE PRIVATE ADDICTION FIELD

Gladstone Lodge is located in a picturesque rural area with a largely white and middle-income population. It runs two separate programs, one for men and one for women. New clients find that the large, two-story, multiwing building does not look fancy—especially the women's unit. The building's siding is old, and the colors are drab. Inside, faux-wood paneling, pictures of old white men, and a large lobby with a fireplace make Gladstone look like a fraternal organization's clubhouse or a ski resort that needs renovation. One client even called the women's unit "a dump." Yet its isolated, bucolic location places the Lodge squarely in the nineteenth-century tradition of sending the errant to rural institutions, far from the corrupting influence of urban life, to foster health and moral reform. There are private homes around the Lodge but no sidewalks, and the nearest town is far away. It would take at least half an hour to walk to the closest commercial establishment, a roadside convenience store. In addition to its potential therapeutic value, isolation aids control. Staff members in the men's program joked to me that they talked up the existence of bears in the woods so the "city boys" wouldn't run off. Following the familial logic underpinning reformatories, Bill and Faye live on the property. Their house is so close that clients take a daily walk right in front of their lawn. Faye and Bill serve as managers, parental figures, and spiritual guides to the twelve steps. Given its setting, approach, and leaders in recovery, it is a classic addiction rehab program.

Both the Lodge and WTS are licensed by the state's Department of Substance Abuse Services.[26] However, the Lodge is a private-pay program, meaning it takes no government funding or public insurance like Medicaid. Thus, it has no formal relationship with the criminal justice or welfare systems. Its customers (staff members call them either "clients" or "patients"—the latter a term never used at WTS) pay with private health insurance or their own money. Because state funding and the penal system are so deeply involved in treatment, private-pay facilities constitute a minority of all rehabs. There is enormous variation in the cost and luxuriousness of private-pay programs. Some charge well above $30,000 a month and offer the look and services of a five-star hotel, including spas, acupuncture treatment, and equine therapy. In comparison, Gladstone Lodge is a modest and inexpensive program that costs $9,000 per month and offers few frills. Nevertheless, with a gym, a pool, and beautiful wooded grounds, it is a far cry from what women like Donisha find at WTS. The men's and women's programs at the Lodge are completely separate, operating in different buildings connected by a hallway. While Bill and Faye manage the whole organization, the two programs are staffed by different counselors. The men's program is about three times bigger than the women's (which is a typical ratio in addiction treatment).[27] In fact, the Lodge could not survive if it offered only a women's program, which with an average of around twelve clients was chronically under its maximum of twenty-four.

Pathways to the Lodge

To get clients, the Lodge contracts with insurance companies, employers, and labor unions (including those for police, steelworkers, steamfitters, utility, sanitation, and health-care workers). This means that a majority of its clients came through the union or employer pathway. Family pressure and resources create a second pathway. A smaller number of women take a third pathway: the state's CPS system. Like some WTS women, they must go to treatment to retain custody of their children. I met only a handful of women who had no institutional or social network connection to the Lodge. They had found the program on the Internet. Work and family operate at three important stages of women's pathways to treatment. First, employers, unions, and family members often propel women to seek treatment in the first place. Second, these networks also recommend the Lodge, as Sarah's doctor colleague did. Finally, they help pay for treatment. While a couple of Lodge clients had criminal cases that drove them to rehab, CPS represents the only pathway the Lodge shares with WTS. Lodge clients never had the threat of prison hanging over their heads. Nevertheless, work-based pathways are not devoid of coercion. Many Lodge women must go to treatment if they want to keep their jobs. Lodge staff called this situation "job jeopardy," and that was what the program ran on. One black member of a utility workers' union told me that she felt like she had been "kidnapped" by her job when they took her to the Lodge, since it all happened so soon after she was caught for using. She barely had time to arrange care for her son. The police union was known for immediately whisking officers into treatment, given the legal problems posed by substance use on the force.

Because of this relationship to workplaces and insurance, the Lodge plays a role in practices of employer discipline and our employment-based system for distributing health care and other social goods. As with many things about addiction treatment, the work pathway started informally. Early on in his career, Bill cultivated relationships with police unions by helping a few officers dry out. These officers began to refer coworkers with drinking problems to Bill, a relationship that was eventually formalized when the Lodge contracted with what are called employee assistance programs (EAPs). These employer-paid benefit programs help workers deal with personal problems that might affect the workplace. While EAPs now help with many kinds of problems, they have their origins in efforts to respond to employee substance abuse. In 1959, the AA-affiliated National Council on Alcoholism launched a campaign to get industry and business to address alcoholism, pointing to how it hurts productivity. The council used the slogan "save the man, save the investment."[28] The Lodge's union ties began with alcoholics, but it claims to be one of the earliest programs to treat drug users along with alcoholics. The move of old-style alcoholism rehabs into drug treatment would not have happened without the growing legitimacy of the idea of addiction. This system of work-based treatment expanded in 1986, during the war on drugs, when President Ronald Reagan required federal workplaces to be drug free. Federal and state governments then implemented widespread testing for employees and contractors. Although the Lodge avoids state funding, it benefits from these regulations.

Families are another major pathway to Gladstone Lodge. Although it is an informal institution of social control, families can push women to go to treatment and fund it. In addition, many women I met had heard of the Lodge through a relative or family friend who had been a client. Work-based coercion can operate through informal mechanisms as well, as it did with Sarah. This happened to Adriana, a Jewish Latina woman in her early forties. She worked as a schoolteacher in a nearby town and was pressed informally into treatment when her principal threatened to fire her for her drinking. Her work-based insurance provided her with more choice than less-privileged people have. Adriana first attended a rehab that took many mandated clients and people on Medicaid, but she found this place "ghetto" and switched to the Lodge. Because most unions are male-dominated, Lodge women are as likely to be a relative of a union member as they are to be a member themselves.[29] In contrast, the men's program contained a much higher proportion of union members. Thus, gendered patterns of employment led the work and family pathways to overlap. Meredith, a middle-aged, British black woman from the city, was able to fund treatment at the Lodge because she had health insurance through her husband, who was a steamfitter. Laughing, Meredith explained to me that even though they were separated, she decided not to divorce him because of how good his insurance was.

These networked pathways and the Lodge's good reputation mean that an enormous number of women I met were what might be called repeat customers. Take Doris, for example. She was a middle-class white woman of around sixty from a suburban area who had been at the Lodge a few years earlier. Much to her embarrassment, she relapsed. Doris was initially propelled into rehab after her son and husband staged an intervention when other ways of trying to control her drinking (such as not allowing her to drive) did not work. She first chose the Lodge because a member of her extended family had been there. Now having "picked up" drinking again, Doris wanted to return because she felt the Lodge was a special place. However, her husband thought that if its methods hadn't worked the first time, there was no reason to try them again. Doris insisted because she blamed her relapse on her failure to "work" the twelve steps properly. Similarly, Stacy, a white woman in her twenties who used heroin, came through family connections and blamed her relapse on herself. Her mother was a close friend of one of the Lodge's founders—they had been in AA together years ago. Stacy was at the Lodge for fourteen months as an "extended" client. The Lodge had a handful of such clients, who help pay for their long stays by working in administrative or therapeutic roles. However, Stacy relapsed a few months after leaving, and her parents paid for her return to the Lodge. These word-of-mouth recommendations are vital to the Lodge's survival, so it cultivates its alumni with newsletters, events, and holiday cards. Mila, a Latina union member, told me that she had been there six months before, following years of sobriety. When she returned, she said the counselors remembered her and hugged her, which made her feel less embarrassed about having to come back. She explained that she had come back to the Lodge because the counselors there "were different" than those in other rehabs.

Gladstone Lodge may not take state funding, but it cannot avoid clients with legal issues. People with CPS cases made up a sizable minority of clients in the women's program, but there were none in the men's. CPS creates an especially gendered pathway to rehab. Moreover, it was often family members who reported women to CPS. Grace was an immigrant from Ireland and a repeat customer at the Lodge, telling me it was her third time in rehab that year. "I do have pending court cases," she said. "I didn't even have a parking ticket until this October!" Grace then explained that she had a car accident while drunk, and her kids had been in the car. This led to a CPS case and a pending driving while intoxicated (DWI) case. After the accident her husband "took an order of protection out against me so I can't be in the house," leaving Grace unable to see her children and without anywhere to turn. The Lodge ended up offering her a substantially reduced rate that staffers call a "scholarship," and she became an extended client who stayed for many months.

For a handful of the women I met during my research at the Lodge, the criminal justice system prompted their entry into treatment. Clustered in the less serious parts of the system, their criminal justice pathways are unlike those that send women to WTS. Most were like Grace and had DWI cases. Staff referred to some people as "mandated" to get treatment when this was not quite accurate. Susan, mentioned in the introduction, was on probation. Despite this, she kept using cocaine. Although probation officials never caught her, using caused trouble with her sober fiancé. Susan voluntarily entered rehab to save her relationship and get her driver's license reissued. Three other women called "mandated" were actually pretrial and hoped to avoid being sentenced to jail time by entering rehab and pleasing the judge in their cases. Only Alexa, a white, middle-class, twenty-year-old heroin user, was mandated to get treatment for something other than DWI—in her case, by probation officials. I never met a Lodge client on parole from prison or mandated by a drug court, but most WTS clients were in one of those categories. Moreover, all Lodge clients with criminal cases had chosen the program themselves and funded rehab with private insurance or self-payment. Alexa had been at a penal rehab before, like a couple of other Lodge women. Her parents' means enabled Alexa to choose the Lodge for her eighth try at treatment. Alexa's ability to choose a nonpenal rehab suggests it is not simply a criminal record that bifurcates the treatment field. Rather, it is the interaction of criminalization with class and racial marginalization.

The Lodge's pathways create a female client population that is mostly white and working- or middle-class. However, the clients had a wider range of ethnic and class backgrounds than I found at WTS. Of the ninety-one women in treatment at the Lodge during my research, about 12 percent were black and about 10 percent were Latina. The rest were white.[30] The women of color tended to be union members from the city. The Lodge draws many clients from the largely white towns and suburbs nearby. In addition, its long-standing relationship with police unions means I met several officers there. It does attract some professional, upper-middle-class women, but overall its clients are usually not wealthy or highly educated. They are, however, more privileged than most working-class people because they have insurance and/or are affiliated with a union. The political scientist Marie Gottschalk called this privatized safety net of insurance and union benefits a "shadow welfare state."[31] Some women I met at the Lodge could have been WTS clients if not for one family member with a good job and a little luck evading the law. For example, Nickie was an eighteen-year-old, working-class, Latina heroin user who lived very near WTS—but her father was a union member. And Sylvia, a middle-aged black woman, had received treatment for crack use at a penal rehab near WTS twenty years earlier. But when she developed a drinking problem later in life, her union job enabled her to cross the divide between rehabs.

Joining the "Fellowship"

Women going to Gladstone Lodge for treatment must be driven to its isolated location. Often the driver is a family member, but some women are picked up by a Lodge driver or an EAP representative. Multiple women at the Lodge told me that they had arrived high or drunk, for "one last time." They notoriously pack too much stuff, and they have to surrender cigarettes, wallets, money, products with alcohol, and mobile phones when they arrive. These items are not permitted at the Lodge and are held in a safe until the women leave. New arrivals see the nursing department staff and have an intake interview with Vincent, a jolly former Lodge client who is the head of admissions and insurance company wrangler. Then new arrivals receive an embossed folder containing information such as the dress code and workbooks to guide their fourth and fifth steps. After that, they head to the women's unit.

The men's and women's programs were kept physically separate, with different staff members and different living, eating, and therapeutic quarters. The women's unit counselors were all female, the men's mostly male. (All staffers were white.) The two groups of counselors worked separately, except for Ruth, the Women's Unit Director, who met with other managers. The staff worked hard to maintain strict gender segregation. Each program separately used shared amenities like the gym. Clients were moved through the facility at different, carefully coordinated times to ensure that men and women did not see one another. If male and female clients ended up in the same space, usually only for special events, they were not allowed to look at each other or communicate in any way. Most rehab programs do not treat men and women separately and few treat only women. In part this is a result of women's smaller numbers, but it is also because the field has been dominated by men and organized around men's experiences with substance abuse.[32] At the Lodge, however, the marginalization of the women's program was palpable. The men's program is the most visible and powerful in the organization. Its staff dominates the managerial and decision-making positions, and its clients have more access to the shared facilities.

While the new women do not know it, they first enter through the men's spaces. The women's program is cloistered in a very cramped wing of the Lodge to maintain the program's strict gender separation. When women enter, they see a spacious living room with large windows, a massive fish tank, and huge stone fireplace. Cushy chairs sit by wood coffee tables that hold chess, checkers, and puzzles. The walls contain photos of Lodge celebrations and oil paintings of desperate drunks. Off the living room is the large, cafeteria-style dining room, with windows; pictures of the Last Supper; a mural of the Lodge's renovation plans; and another enormous, unused fireplace. To the left is a chapel with stained-glass windows and the men's residential units. To the right is the women's wing. Compared to the men's comfortable, airy spaces, the women's unit is tiny and considerably less well appointed.

Moving from the men's space to the women's was a significant experience for new clients because the women's space is so much less impressive. To get to there, you exit the men's living room, going past a standing barrier screen, which is there to prevent visual contact between male and female clients. Women then enter a tiny lobby with a comparatively tiny fish tank, two chairs, framed inspirational sayings about women and sobriety, a photo of Faye's mother, and a table with pamphlets that no one looks at. The lobby leads to a long corridor that contains staff members' offices and clients' bedrooms, as well as a laundry room and a bank of pay phones. Women sleep three per room; each woman has a twin bed and a dresser. Every room has a bathroom. The unit has only two public rooms, which in familial fashion are called the kitchen and the living room. The living room is cluttered but homey, with small windows, two couches, a piano, a TV, board games, a poster of the twelve steps, and many decorations. This is where most therapeutic groups are held. Above the door leading out of the living room is a sign stating, "Leave It on the Mountain." The kitchen is actually a dining room with cafeteria tables; a soda vending machine; and a supply of coffee, tea, bread, and condiments. It contains a sign that demands clients sit at meals for thirty minutes before getting up and that bans reading to encourage conversation, imploring, "help maintain the art of dining."

This emphasis on connecting with other clients is key to treatment. Gladstone Lodge aims to recreate the bonding and camaraderie that twelve-step groups call fellowship. Lodge staff members refer to clients collectively as "the fellowship." The women's fellowship is symbolized through a painting in the unit's lobby titled *The Work*. It depicts one young white woman giving AA's main text (commonly called the Big Book) to another young white woman who is lying on the ground surrounded by liquor bottles. Like the women in the painting, clients were supposed to reach out to each other as part of "the work" of recovery. This was institutionalized via rotating client positions.

One of the weekly roles was the Greeter, who had the responsibility to meet new clients, show them around, explain the rules, and spend time with them in their first days. This helped to integrate new women into the fellowship. Other weekly positions of authority were the Mayor, who woke everyone in the morning and watched the staff perform a daily "room check" with the Deputy, who also announced group sessions and took attendance. Finally, the Go-Get-Her retrieved late clients for group. The rest of the positions involved chores like cleaning the dining tables, vacuuming the living room, and monitoring the pay phones during the time clients were allowed to get and receive calls. Unlike at WTS, the chores rotated and were not used as punishments.

Every woman at the Lodge has the same schedule, and all clients are in the groups. Each day begins with a meditation, followed by a therapeutic group, lunch, a group devoted to one of the twelve steps, an extended time off, and finally an afternoon group. After the therapeutic day is over, the women eat, do one more meditation, and are free to do crafts, watch one of the few movies the Lodge has on DVD, or write in their workbooks. Individual counseling sessions happen weekly in between these activities. This schedule gives women a lot of down time. As long as the men are not there and a staff member is around to supervise, women may use the Lodge's other facilities during this time. They can go to the gym or the bright and airy place called the "sun room" to buy candy with money they withdraw from cash deposited with the program. However, to keep clients focused on recovery, they are not allowed to have any outside entertainment—no books, TV, or music. The only books permitted are Lodge-approved recovery texts. Clients' only connection to the outside world comes through daily newspapers that they can buy. Clients are not allowed to leave the Lodge, but they can take twice-daily walks outside on the facility's grounds. They may call family members each day, but only for five minutes at a time. Such cloistering very much reflects the tradition of moral treatment and total institutions. As this description suggests, the Lodge is not a hospital setting, nor is its treatment method medicalized. Indeed, its staff members are substance abuse counselors who are almost all former addicts or alcoholics. There were a couple of nurses on the staff and one social worker (also in recovery), but a doctor visited only once a week. The program's twelve-step commitment to total abstinence made staff members reluctant to administer psychiatric prescription drugs. Even through medicalized techniques and professionals did not play a large role in the program, the health insurance system did.

A Medical Reason: The Limits of the Health-Care Model

Health-care-based funding had major implications for the structure of Gladstone Lodge's program and its viability as a business. I initially guessed that the Lodge would offer a wider range of services than WTS because it was not reliant on public funding and competed to attract customers in an increasingly luxury-oriented industry. However, this was not the case. Private-pay programs cannot maintain the same structure or range of services as do penal rehabs. This is because insurance companies will not pay for more than one month of treatment, nor do they cover ancillary services. As a result, most women at the Lodge stay for twenty-eight days. Insurance coverage for addiction treatment was never generous, but with the advent of managed care in the 1990s it has become increasingly limited. It will not cover residential programs unless individuals have failed in outpatient treatment, sometimes several times. Individuals must pay for longer stays themselves. Vincent claimed that clients once got forty-two days, but now they are lucky to get over fourteen. Every extra day must be justified by a "medical reason." Insurance time limits and paperwork requirements produce enormous hassles for the Lodge staff. Every two days the counselors must file reports with insurance companies to explain the clients' progress. Staff members found this only enabled them to cut off coverage. Vincent told me he constantly fights for more time, using every conceivable "medical reason"—including high blood pressure, family conflicts, and even pending court cases. I saw restrictive coverage force many women to leave sooner than they wanted. Other clients spent each day wondering if they would have to leave. One of the program's responses was to offer scholarships to extend the treatment, but this cut into the organization's revenue. It was, at best, a stop-gap measure.

Everyone at the Lodge hated insurance companies. They were the target of constant derision. The uncertainty of insurance coverage forced the staff to constantly recalibrate individual treatment plans, which was enormously difficult. At one case review meeting, I heard Ruth happily announce that Amy was "getting one more week." This was greeted with cheers and applause from the other counselors and optimistic proclamations about how much she would benefit from the extra time. A lively and quick Jewish woman in her fifties, Ruth was delighted that they had recently been able to get two women twenty-one days when they originally had only two weeks. But she announced that another managed care company was getting stricter: "now they want you to fail in outpatient twice" before paying for inpatient treatment, she reported. Joan, a counselor reacted with a dismayed gasp. While Ruth wrote these updates in the women's charts, she noted that "now we have issues with Liz." They would have to wait to hear whether she would be leaving in a couple of days or not. The state requires an after-care plan, but compared to WTS, there is little the Lodge can do after women leave. Instead, insurance companies (and thus the Lodge) rely largely on twelve-step groups. Departing clients are told to attend a Narcotics or Alcoholics Anonymous meeting that day and every day for the next ninety days. However, unions reduce clients' vulnerability by providing extra support. EAP representatives talked regularly with the counselors and were thus able to coordinate after care. The representatives drove union clients straight to a twelve-step meeting in their neighborhood after their discharge from the Lodge. Most unions also maintained funds for addiction treatment that could cover what insurance did not.[33] This means that unionized clients often stayed longer than those relying only on insurance or self-payment.

Because of insurance constraints, the Lodge struggled to get enough clients—especially in the women's program. This was made even more difficult by a new state law that prohibited smoking anywhere at rehabilitation facilities, which caused many people to go out of state for treatment. Lodge staff members told me that volume was down at rehabs throughout the state. The smoking ban changed the day-to-day culture at the Lodge. Bill and Faye decided that they had to treat cigarettes like any other substance and asked the staff to refrain from smoking until after work. In addition, the Lodge forbids client smoke breaks. Susan, who was a repeat customer, claimed that before the ban clients bonded more tightly because they had regular staff-free moments to talk. Thus, clients had to quit both their "drug of choice" and smoking at the same time, which caused the staff never-ending control problems and a sequence of major conflicts about clients' sneaking cigarettes. This reveals the power of state agendas to shape Gladstone Lodge, despite it being a private-pay program. Nevertheless, the state and therefore the racial and gender politics of drugs play a larger role at WTS.

Women's Treatment Services, Punishment, and Welfare

"This is not the Betty Ford Clinic," declared WTS's deputy director at our first meeting in 2004. Indeed, it is not. WTS is an intensive residential treatment facility for women that serves as an alternative to incarceration. The fact that she started out by distinguishing WTS from upscale private-pay rehabs was far more telling than I realized at the time. WTS refers to the women it treats as "clients," just as Gladstone Lodge staff members do, but for WTS women their only other choice is usually incarceration. Like most penal rehabs, WTS is a nonprofit organization funded by the city, state, and federal governments as a correctional program located in what is euphemistically called "the community." For WTS that means a deserted, run-down block in a low-income black and Latino neighborhood. The block has an imposing public school at one end and a dingy convenience store at the other, outside of which I regularly observed a handful of drug dealers. Instead of insurance and workplaces, it is criminal justice institutions that shape its treatment program, who is sent there, and what rehab entails. Not only do private-pay and penal rehabs treat different populations, but they also offer different services and rely on different forms of power. As the coming chapters will show, this has significant consequences for how the programs define and treat addiction.

WTS would not exist without the penal state's support for addiction treatment through both the criminal justice and welfare systems. The expansion of treatment in the 1970s created the first programs to divert people with drug problems from jail into community-based treatment.[34] This fit with the rehabilitative ideal of the time, but mandated treatment grew again during the punitive turn, pumping money and people into places like WTS. As a result, addiction treatment is more deeply entangled with the penal and welfare state than it is with the health-care system.[35] Drug courts are major funders and shape penal treatment methods, instituting a preference for confrontational therapy, life-skills training, and the liberal use of jail time to coerce compliance. Privately run, community-based penal rehabs are the centerpiece of efforts to reduce incarceration and a key site for governing through addiction. While the criminal justice system mandates people to go to various levels of treatment, including outpatient counseling, I found that intensive residential facilities like WTS are always entangled with punishment and welfare provision. This makes them unlike inpatient rehabs such as the Lodge, which can operate outside the penal state.

Parole and drug courts are WTS's largest sources of funding. But WTS also works with state poverty management and social service agencies, most notably Temporary Assistance to Needy Families (TANF), as well as CPS and family courts. WTS cobbles together funding from several other sources, including Medicaid, the state's Department of Substance Abuse Services, the city's office for homeless services, federal grants, and private donations. The women who arrive at WTS also come with dollars attached to them. WTS enrolls each woman in whatever public assistance programs she is eligible for. Then it takes what WTS calls a "rent" out of this money and saves the rest for clients, who can access it only as a reward for doing well in the program and rising through the four stages of treatment. With this byzantine combination of funds, WTS is able to offer substance abuse treatment at little cost to women, including those without health insurance. However, women cannot easily access this treatment without being criminalized.

Pathways to WTS

WTS's role in penal and welfare state institutions makes the program part of our systems for managing both crime and poverty, producing three main pathways to WTS: parole, criminal courts, and CPS. Nearly all of the approximately fifty women that WTS could house at any one time were mandated to treatment there by the criminal justice system or pushed into treatment by CPS.[36] Based on my observations, parole and drug courts refer a large majority of the clients, but so do traditional criminal courts and probation officials. Court-mandated clients are diverted to rehab in lieu of incarceration, and parolees have recently left prison. If women do not comply or "abscond," they can be referred back to parole or court and end up incarcerated. Criminal justice institutions pay for longer treatment stays than do health insurance companies, making WTS one of the most restrictive kinds of rehab. Women like Donisha, a CPS client, and Christine, the drug court client in the introduction, go to WTS's largest (with about thirty to forty women) and longest (nine to twelve months) "alternative to incarceration" (ATI) stream, referred to as the Residential Program. ATI clients are often nonviolent offenders, convicted of their first felony charge, or women paroled from prison for the first time. Most other parolees come to WTS's three-to-six-month Restabilization Program (which is also residential, in that clients live there) because they have violated the conditions of their parole. The Residential and Restabilization Programs do much of their treatment together, but restabilization clients have more privileges; live in more autonomous, single-room-occupancy-style housing next door to the main building; and have more freedom to leave and to prepare their own food.

Roxanne was paroled to WTS. A white heroin user nearing forty, she spent a few unhappy months in the Restabilization Program, where she was bullied by other clients and dissatisfied with her counselor, and was finally given a pass to see her family. While out on the pass, Roxanne relapsed with alcohol and ended up in the hospital with alcohol poisoning. Instead of reincarcerating Roxanne, her parole officer and WTS agreed to move her to the Residential Program, starting her six months all over again and entering at the beginning orientation level. Roxanne was upset about the extra time away from her children and husband, but she preferred to be in the Residential Program because she had made friends with women there. When Roxanne successfully completed the program, she became what WTS and drug courts call, in an effort to distinguish what they do from prison, a graduate. Roxanne was even able to walk across a stage at WTS's elaborate graduation ceremony. Nevertheless, she had to attend WTS's after-care program at least three times a week for an additional six months, making it hard for her to move to another area or work long hours. Roxanne's transfer shows that clients' placement depended on how both WTS and criminal justice officials interpret women's needs. She had much less choice than Lodge clients did.

The fact that Donisha ended up at WTS with Roxanne and Christine shows that the criminal justice and child welfare systems both govern through addiction, using the same institutions. A classic part of the welfare state, CPS is

designed to help children at risk of neglect and abuse by regulating and providing services to families. Drugs are a major target of these agencies. Jennifer
Reich's study of child welfare agencies in California found that 80 percent
of cases were drug related. The use of drugs, even marijuana, was "indisput-
ably the greatest factor in considering parental ability."[37] Other individuals get
involved with CPS through being arrested or incarcerated, which can lead to
loss of custody. Most commonly, it is mothers who come under CPS's purview because they are typically responsible for child care, and state authorities
hold mothers to higher standards than they do fathers.[38] CPS agencies also
disproportionately target African American women.[39] Because of the panic
over crack babies, hospitals now test women giving birth like Donisha and
refer those who test positive to CPS agencies. While CPS stipulations are not
technically a criminal sanction, the racial and gender politics of the punitive
turn are at the heart of these practices. As a result, many women come to WTS
because of both CPS and criminal cases. They risk losing their parental rights
and going to prison if they do poorly at WTS.

As a result of these pathways, WTS women reflect the penal system's disproportionately low-income and nonwhite population. About 70 percent of
the program's clients are African American, while 20 percent are Latina and
10 percent are white.[40] Although there is some variation, WTS women typically have very low incomes, with limited work and educational histories.
About three-quarters of the women are mothers. WTS reports that about
80-90 percent of its clients have histories of sexual or domestic abuse. This
is not unusual for women who have been in prison. The various pathways
to WTS mean that its clients had a range of life experiences—some were
quite new to being criminalized—but most women's lives had been marked
by interactions with what Susan Sered and Maureen Norton-Hawk call "the
circuit" of programs, jails, homeless shelters, halfway homes, welfare offices,
and hospitals that regulate poor women.[41] This loose network of agencies
makes up the bottom of the social safety net in the United States. Like welfare reform, these institutions focus more on disciplining behavior than on
providing resources to the needy. Thus, the women in Sered and Norton-
Hawk's study were shuttled around, trapped by contradictory or impossible
expectations, and ended up no better off than they had been initially. The
criminal justice system and CPS play key roles in this circuit and render
rehab one of its core institutions.

WTS was deeply embedded in the circuit. Indeed, it had many clients who had spent their lives cycling in and out of foster care, group homes,
juvenile detention, and mental institutions—finally landing in prison, at which
point WTS stepped in. One of my first jobs as a volunteer at WTS was to
call Medicaid-funded detoxification centers to get them to refer clients to the

program. To help increase admissions, I designed a pamphlet advertising WTS's small outpatient program for women who had a home approved by the criminal justice system. The Restabilization Program's director, Patricia—a black and Latina woman—told me that the pamphlet should emphasize that women did not need health insurance. After completing that project, I called homeless shelters, halfway houses, and single-room-occupancy facilities to find homes for WTS's graduating clients. Housing for women with drug convictions, especially those who have children, is not easy to find. As a result, many WTS graduates ended up in other addiction-related institutions, such as sober homes or halfway houses, because there are not many other options.

The rehab a person ends up in has surprisingly little to do with her substance abuse. Many WTS women had long histories of heavy drug use, but some did not. For instance, one young mother mandated to WTS was an occasional marijuana smoker, but she did not use other drugs. A neighbor with whom she had a prior disagreement called the police on her after smelling marijuana coming from her apartment. The woman was mandated to WTS for one year, and the state placed her two children in foster care. Gladstone Lodge had more alcohol and prescription drug users than WTS did, but the Lodge had plenty of illegal drug users too. In fact, national data suggest that people sent to treatment by the criminal justice system may have less severe substance use issues than the people who voluntarily enter programs like Gladstone Lodge. Mandated clients have fewer previous episodes of treatment and are more likely to have alcohol or marijuana as their primary substance of abuse than harder drugs like heroin or cocaine.[42] Several studies of mandated treatment programs have found that a significant number of clients are drug dealers with only minimal histories of drug use.[43] What this means is that although WTS clients overall had lower socioeconomic status than Lodge clients, they did not necessarily have worse substance abuse problems.

The intensity of the treatment program to which a person is sent can say as much about her economic neediness and social marginalization as it does about the severity of her substance use. Drug court case managers, parole officers, intake staff, and others use a state-required clinical tool to determine the level of care each individual needs. According to this tool, what distinguishes people in need of "intensive residential treatment" at facilities like WTS from those in need of "inpatient rehabilitation" programs such as the Lodge are significant deficits in everyday functioning or social skills, isolation from conventional social relations, and inappropriate behavior. In practice these criteria reflect the interrelated traits of poverty, racial marginalization, and criminalization, which then ultimately structure individuals' pathways to treatment. Penal officials' clinical decisions take into account a woman's family supports, her financial situation, and her history of sexual victimization. Based on the state's own criteria for placement, having a low income or limited education are in themselves risk factors for recidivism and relapse, that signal need for an intensive residential program. So, for example, some WTS women were mandated by parole officials because of a positive drug test, but many parolees were mandated to WTS because they had a personal crisis—such as becoming homeless, losing a job, or fleeing domestic violence—that made them unable to meet their parole stipulations. The requirement that people under correctional supervision reside at a known address, combined with a vulnerable population and an inadequate social safety net, means that penal rehabs are one of the few places where officials can secure housing and services for the poor. Patricia told me that most WTS clients would be homeless if they did not reside at the facility. Consequently, many women come to a place like WTS because they have nowhere else to go. Thus, WTS is both a penal institution and a social welfare provider. Its role reveals that drug war policies both deny welfare support (such as eligibility for public housing) to people with drug convictions and simultaneously link them with rehab-based welfare supports through criminalization. This renders addiction treatment a solution to social problems that the penal system both creates and is expected to manage.

Like previous iterations of the welfare state, the rehab safety net is profoundly gendered. The central ideology animating WTS's version of penal-welfare is known as women-centered or gender-responsive treatment. This approach to treatment emerged from recovery culture and is increasingly popular in the penal system. Advocates of gender-responsive treatment claim it addresses women's unique needs. In keeping with this model, WTS offers parenting classes, trauma therapy, domestic violence education, and family therapy in addition to substance abuse counseling and assistance securing housing, education, and employment. Its women-centered approach cultivated a reputation, client base, and state grants targeted at women. TANF money funded family services that taught women to maintain proper households so they could regain custody of their children. Yvonne, the legal services director at WTS, told me that parole officers and judges often refer a woman to WTS rather than to a mixed-sex program when they have reason to think she has some gendered problem, such as having a history of sexual abuse or a CPS case. These gendered services appeal to some women: Yvonne showed me letters from incarcerated women asking for admission to the program. They were handwritten and sounded desperate; many expressed interest in the women-only environment.

Gladstone Lodge also billed itself as women-centered, but this treatment model is primarily used by penal programs.[44] Rehabs exclusively serving women belong almost entirely to the publicly funded arena, relying less on private health insurance or self-payment.[45] I suggest that this pattern is due to two factors: women's lesser access to good employment and the policy impact of racialized moral panics over women's substance use. Separate lines of state funding have existed for women's treatment since the 1970s, but they were greatly expanded in response to the crack-baby panic. This opened the door for women from the recovery movement to petition the state to institute gender-sensitive programs.[46] However, the availability of these services is subject to political will. During my fieldwork, TANF funding was cut, and a WTS staff member with the title of activities of daily living specialist was laid off. Her work had focused on socializing clients by teaching them basic practical and social skills—everything from hygiene, etiquette, and budgeting to a group called current events. Marcus, the Residential Program director, who was a middle-aged black man, blamed this on the economy and President George W. Bush. Gender-responsive treatment has gained traction in the years since. Eventually, the state decided that all eligible women in prison originally from WTS's neighborhood would be paroled to the program.

Rehabs like WTS are a form of social provision overlooked by scholars of the welfare state. Thus, the state uses rehab to manage racial, class, and gender marginalization. WTS links women up with more social services than they could receive from any other organization or social program. Because of its women-centered strategy, it even offers more services than most penal rehabs.[47] However, it also means that the state places incredibly complex social problems like gender violence, poverty, and homelessness in the collective lap of WTS staff members. And for a woman in need, access to these services requires being criminalized and, thus, losing basic rights. Mandated treatment signals the reemergence of some aspects of rehabilitative penal-welfarism, but this form of punishment is organized according to a new logic: addiction.

WTS as a Penal Satellite

WTS positions itself as an antidote to the unjust treatment of low-income women of color. Regardless, it must operate within the criminal justice system. Lynne Haney links privately run, publicly funded penal programs like WTS to neoliberal changes in the state, such as privatization and decentralization. These agencies open the door to new modes of governance, but they are still satellites of the state.[48] While Gladstone Lodge is part of workplace and familial discipline, WTS's authority relies on a dense web of gendered and racialized penal tactics, including policing that targets low-level offenses, drug testing parolees, and the removal of newborns from drug-using mothers. In line with these tactics, WTS carries out key aspects of punishment. Every month WTS reports on its clients to courts and parole officers. I barely saw Jay, a young black man who was WTS's court liaison. He seemed to spend every minute of the day running from one courthouse to another, reporting on clients. WTS's reporting duties mean that its staff engages in near-constant surveillance of clients, including administering random drug tests. I would often walk by rubber-gloved staff members standing in the hallway in front of an open bathroom door watching a woman urinate. Not surprisingly, this is an awkward experience for many women, including one who, surrounded by people talking in the corridor, asked Karen, a counselor, to turn on the faucet to make it easier for her to go. Such practices reveal WTS's role as a penal institution. If a woman breaks important rules or has "dirty urine," WTS reports this to legal officials. The woman then faces sanctions, referred to as being "on contract," or expulsion. And if a woman absconds, a warrant is issued for her arrest.

Yvonne, an outgoing and sharp-witted black woman, ran WTS's Legal Services Department and dealt with the criminal justice system. She made it clear that the state also constrained WTS. Her department screened potential clients; made the monthly reports to parole officers, judges, and family court; and sent Jay to clients' numerous hearings. They always seemed to be scrambling to keep up with outside agencies' expectations while also fulfilling their responsibilities to manage clients' social, psychological, and economic issues. One day I walked into WTS and found Yvonne sitting at her computer, surrounded by precariously tall stacks of files and looking stressed out. Apparently a previous employee had done a bad job of gathering data and keeping records, and WTS had supplied parole with the wrong discharge dates for an unknown number of clients. Yvonne was now trying to correct the problem. She looked me in the eye and noted seriously that WTS could lose millions of dollars; the parole system is their biggest contract.

Like Gladstone Lodge, WTS needs a constant stream of clients to sustain itself, and staff members had to hustle to make sure it remained on criminal justice officials' radar. One day I saw Ayana, a black woman around thirty who was the intake specialist, discuss leaving WTS with a client who had arrived the night before for the Residential Program. The client was a young black woman in her early twenties. She was crying and claimed that she needed day treatment, not a residential program; she couldn't handle being there. Unlike those who had been on "the circuit," this woman had never been in a program like WTS. Ayana called the client's parole officer on speakerphone, and they worked together to convince the woman that it was normal to be scared at first. The client refused to change her mind and insisted that she did not want to stay and could live with her family. Eventually the officer agreed to find her day treatment and parole her to her family's address. Moments after she left to get her things, Patricia learned that the woman was leaving WTS and got mad at Ayana, saying, "We have day treatment! Why didn't she tell them that?" Frantic, Patricia bolted off to inform the departing client about the program's other offerings.

WTS staffers must figure out how to combine control with the program's therapeutic and welfarist aims. This is not an easy task, as later chapters will show. Because of WTS's ties to different welfare and criminal justice agencies, counselors juggle multiple treatment timelines, rules, and goals. While drug courts are known for sharing the program's emphasis on therapeutic accomplishments, other agencies stress drug test results and whether clients commit another crime. They use drug tests and recidivism not only to measure clients' progress, but also to assess WTS's success. I found that state criminal justice officials typically deferred to WTS's decisions about clients' length of stay, discharge dates, and indications of progress. However, WTS depended on the state's power to punish for its leverage over clients. Occasionally the authorities even released women from their mandates before WTS thought they were ready.

One of the bigger crises during my fieldwork at WTS occurred when a client had gone for a month without taking her psychiatric medication, and no one had noticed. At the weekly staff meeting, Marcus harshly criticized the counselors. He and Patricia emphasized that this was an enormous failure of responsibility on WTS's part. Marcus lectured the staffers about their lack of communication: if they had been better at surveillance and shared more information among themselves, they would have been able to piece things together. To WTS's embarrassment, it was the client's parole officer who figured out what had happened. Marcus then offered suggestions about how to facilitate information sharing among staff. Gesticulating wildly and getting increasingly upset, he returned again and again to the refrain, "We are a treatment facility!" His underlings sat quietly, looking uncomfortable. Marcus then demeaned staffers' professionalism by mocking how they doted on the only pregnant client. "Aww, you had a baby," he mimicked in a high-pitched imitation of a woman's voice. He then pointed out that with lower caseloads than staff members at other programs, they had it good, so they should be able to handle their clients. Marcus rhetorically asked how this incident would look to parole. He explained that it would "alienate referral sources." They will "wonder what kind of treatment center this is" and will think WTS is incompetent. They won't send referrals. "No funders mean no jobs and no [WTS]," he said, threateningly. Marcus informed the staff that his boss—WTS's executive director, who worked offsite and had little to do with daily affairs—had called him to ask, "Who lost their job because of this?" As a result of the pressure to demonstrate "success," WTS often discharged women whom staffers saw as difficult or resistant. I could not get data on completion rates for the years I conducted ethnographic research at WTS or on all the clients from the various pathways combined, but completion rates for ATI admissions in 2008 were 63-80 percent. Yet 20-50 percent of admitted clients had administrative discharges and thus were excluded from completion rates. These completion rates are pretty typical compared to similar programs, but the discharge rates are high.

Joining "the House"

Despite being a penal institution, WTS does not look like a prison. There are no guards or imposing fences, just an unlocked wrought-iron gate and a door. You must be buzzed into the three-story building, but anyone can walk out. Inside, WTS feels institutional and run down, with linoleum floors, crowded offices, and old equipment. The front entrance leads directly into the central hallway, which is framed by reception and the intake office. That floor contains the main meeting room, which was the nuns' former chapel; its altar is partially intact and stacked with board games. In addition, there is a cafeteria-style dining room with several circular tables and a kitchen, where a cook works during the day. As part of their chores and punishments, clients prepare dinner for what was called "the house" at night. The basement contains a series of crowded, windowless staff offices, the laundry room, and a small computer lab. On the upper floors are two of the nicer staff offices and residents' bedrooms. Most women live two to four to a room, each of which contains bunk beds and a sink. The women share a bathroom with the other occupants on the floor. Clients must keep their rooms neat and their beds made. Newly admitted women sleep in a very public room called "the dorm," which contains five bunk beds, a staff office, a small library, and a couch. At first, the name "dorm" puzzled me because it seemed like the regular rooms more closely resembled a college dorm, but I realized the name refers to a particular form of prison architecture in which inmates are housed in large rooms with rows of bunk beds. This confusion reveals how my more privileged background gave me a different frame of reference for institutional living. Moreover, WTS's use of prison terminology shows its roots in the penal system.

WTS's busy, informal atmosphere can be alternately warm and intimidating. Newly admitted women walk into a bustling scene that sometimes feels chaotic. Clients come and go, and staff members run back and forth. Unlike at Gladstone Lodge, clients have individualized schedules, and multiple therapeutic groups occur at once. These sessions structure the day and create regular flows of women from room to room. Each client who enters has her belongings searched by the receptionist, who also answers calls, takes deliveries, and dispenses medication. Several times a day, women line up against the wall of the main hallway with plastic cups of water to receive their often-copious quantities of medication. All this activity is pierced by the receptionist's regular announcements over the public address system to the staff and clients (whom she always calls "ladies") about phone calls, visitors, and scheduled smoking breaks. Clients had mixed responses to the place that were framed by their past experiences. The woman who transferred said she could not take WTS, but Ella, a black woman around forty, told me it was "like the Hilton" to her because she had just been incarcerated. Ella noted: "I've got to be here, but I need it. . . . I'm not doing them a favor, they doing me a favor." A more critical client, Lisette, who was Latina and in her thirties, called the place "unprofessional" and "bootleg" for having no nurse or psychiatrist on staff to help with her mental illness. She claimed that WTS was interested only in money and cited the "rent" it took from clients' benefits, suggesting that it was collecting the interest off clients' savings. Lisette thought it was bootleg, but WTS resembles the semiprofessionalization of the Lodge and most rehabs. Its only counselors with advanced degrees were a social worker and a family therapist, both white women. Otherwise, most staff members were state-licensed substance abuse counselors, and they were predominantly black or Latina women. I suspect that like the Lodge counselors, many were in recovery themselves, but they were less open about it.

WTS shares some, but not all, of the features of what Erving Goffman famously called total institutions. In such places, which include prisons, mental institutions, and convents, groups of people live entirely under the institutions' regimented routines, usually with little privacy. While they may seem different, these institutions share disciplinary routines and, importantly, have the power to define their inmates' entire identity. Unlike in regular life, where people have multiple identities such as parent and employee, inmates in total institutions are permitted none of the separation of roles that undergird our sense of self. For Goffman, total institutions are "forcing houses" for transforming people's selves.[49] At WTS, women conduct nearly all of their lives within the institution, living according to a rigid timetable and under constant surveillance. While WTS clients are in treatment for much longer than Lodge clients, they have the ability to leave and thus mitigate the isolation of treatment. As they progress through the levels of treatment, they can get passes to leave for work, to visit family, or to go shopping. This is part of WTS's correctional goal of reintegrating offenders into society. Initially, women are "escorted" by a more senior client, who is expected to report any "deviations" to the staff. Like the Lodge, WTS constrains clients' contact with the outside world. Visits with family and even telephone calls require staff permission, and they are forbidden until clients complete the orientation level.

WTS permits more individuation than most total institutions do, but only when it is aligned with the program's ideology. Women are not required to wear uniforms, but as we will see, how they dress is subject to guidance and regulation. Women decorate their rooms with family photos, stuffed animals, beauty products, and pictures from magazines. If women acquire what counselors determine to be too much stuff, it will be removed. Unlike prisons but like other rehab programs, WTS uses the twelve-step form of address: first name and last initial, such as Donisha S. Staff members go by their first name, a few with the honorific Miss in front. Staffers' decorations emphasize WTS's differences from the prison and its women-centered mission. Throughout the building, posters sporting motivational sayings, the twelve steps, and images of famous black women adorn the walls. These decorations are intended to be inspirational, and their self-help tone is mirrored in the signs and poems women put on their bedroom doors.

Some of the staff offices signal overtly political versions of empowerment. African art gave the professional-looking office of Tabitha, the deputy director, a link to black activism. Although she had little to do with clinical work, Tabitha was the highest-ranking administrator on site and helped set the tone. Patricia could be hard on the clients, but her office contained a poster advocating the reform of state drug laws and another encouraging African Americans to vote. Down the hall from Patricia's office was the office of Margaret, the social worker, and Karen, the family therapist. Their posters emphasized feminist activism, including one for a "Take Back the Night" march against sexual violence. However, these challenges to the system were more prominent on the walls than in the treatment process. In this, as in all other things, WTS blends dynamics of punishment with aspects of recovery culture.

CONCLUSION

This chapter has shown that while addiction treatments have always been stratified, today rehab is bifurcated. In large part, this is a result of how the punitive turn expanded support for legally mandated treatment. Gendered and racialized processes of criminalization interact with class inequality, especially around access to good jobs with benefits. These processes send women to different rehabs with divergent structures and services. Both WTS and Gladstone Lodge rely on the way state and private actors govern through addiction. Yet mapping the pathways to these two programs reveals distinct systems for regulating marginalized populations and those with more privilege. This complicated web of governing institutions, networks, and power relationships reinforces prevailing patterns of social inequality. As a result, WTS and Lodge clients were differently positioned within the institutional power structure at each program. The Lodge's pathways reveal the contours of a private and often informal system that governs through addiction. Surprisingly, this results in less treatment for the more privileged. Indeed, the American criminal justice system appears to be far more generous with rehab than the American healthcare system is. As later chapters will show, the short treatment stays and lack of ancillary services has significant consequences for the kind of treatment the Lodge offers.

Meanwhile, the penal state operates an almost completely separate treatment system. Most research on the punishment emphasizes race. However, I reveal the additional importance of class—in particular, the distinction between the poor and those members of the working class with better jobs. For example, women came to both WTS and the Lodge from the CPS pathway. What determined where they ended up was whether or not they had access to private insurance or cash to pay for treatment. Sylvia's upward mobility to a unionized job enabled her to move from a penal rehab in her youth to the Lodge. Nickie, a working-class, Latina woman involved with crime, probably managed to escape a penal rehab only because of her dad's unionized job. Noncriminal justice funding for treatment, including Medicaid, is often entangled with penal rehabs. Without decent insurance, Nickie would have had to go to a place like WTS, even if she wasn't officially charged with a crime. She would therefore have become criminalized by proxy. As unionization declines, such stories will become increasingly unlikely. With the expansion of penal treatment, more organizations like WTS will sit at the boundary between criminal justice and addiction treatment. In them, new types of punishment are being forged.

CHAPTER 2

Women's Treatment Services

ADDICTED TO PUNISHMENT

EVERY WEDNESDAY AFTERNOON, Women's Treatment Services (WTS) staff members gather for a case review meeting to discuss clients' progress and plan their treatment. The primary, vocational, and after-care counselors join the social worker, family therapist, and two program directors in a small, stuffy, basement room that also serves as WTS's computer lab. Surrounded by ancient, donated computers that barely work, the staff members sit at a conference table, eat lunch, joke, chat, and hunker down for a marathon, three-hour-plus meeting during which they meticulously review what has been happening with the women legally mandated to WTS for addiction treatment. During one of these meetings the staff discussed Sofia, who was two months shy of finishing her nine-month stint at WTS. She seemed to be doing well. She had not relapsed, she had a job, and she even had business cards—much to her counselor's surprise. Because of these accomplishments her parole officer evaluated her and determined that she did not need more treatment. With an early discharge approved, Sofia was free to go. She was eager to leave and requested that WTS also allow her to graduate early.

The assembled staff members were not impressed by Sofia's job or sobriety. In fact, they were upset about the whole situation. For one thing, they thought she was being "cocky." Then Marcus, the director of WTS's Residential Program, added indignantly that when parole refers a woman to WTS, they refer her to the program's standards of treatment. The group speculated about why Sofia would have been granted an early discharge. The staffers finally concluded that Sofia must have "manipulated" her parole officer, rendering the officer blind to her real problems. WTS staffers were perennially concerned that clients were manipulative or cocky, behavior that was viewed as signs of addiction. Sofia was therefore clearly in need of more treatment. Marcus stated that Sofia's "cockiness" was the first sign of an impending relapse. Patricia, the director of the Restabilization Program, started lecturing the counselors about the lesson they should draw from this situation. "Women do need to be empowered," she explained, but "empowerment needs to come later in treatment." Otherwise, clients like Sofia will think they are "ready before they really are." In the end, the staff decided that if Sofia left, WTS would treat her as if she had failed the program. Just like the women parole officers send back to prison for being unsuccessful, Sofia would not be eligible for any after-care services, which include counseling and help finding housing. Patricia noted that Sofia would also not be able to participate in WTS's graduation ceremony, join the alumnae network, or attend alumnae events. Once she "walks out that door," Patricia said, she can never come back.

Sofia could have been a success story. She followed the law. She was not using drugs. By working, Sofia met the official goals of both parole and WTS. Moreover, she was living up to widespread norms about how the poor should act and what it means to be a responsible, independent citizen. Yet WTS staffers did not take her early release, sobriety, and employment as signs that the program had worked or that they were good at their jobs—just the opposite. When Marcus worried about her relapsing, he saw her actions as a sign of dependence, not independence. Although WTS promotes itself as an agency devoted to "empowering" women to "reclaim their lives," Patricia claimed her colleagues had erred by empowering Sofia too much. WTS's take on Sofia is particularly notable because correctional institutions have traditionally used employment and abstinence as indicators of success. Why, then, was Sofia a failure? The staff members felt that she was because they do not think that drug abuse, unemployment, criminal behavior, or laziness are the clients' real problems. Instead, WTS defines addiction as having a weak and dependent self. Consequently, "working on the self" is what indicates success. In these long meetings, WTS staffers spent surprisingly little time discussing women's substance use and criminal behavior. While they expected clients to go through vocational counseling, they did not focus their energy on making clients economically self-sufficient. Sofia's parole officer may have valued sobriety and employment, but WTS took a different approach.

At WTS's 2005 graduation ceremony, the official program distributed to the graduates, family, and friends contained an effusive message from the executive director. She wrote, "We're in the business of helping people overcome their addiction to pain and punishment." For WTS, then, addiction is much bigger than substance abuse. It is a disorder of the whole self, and it acts as a totalizing explanation for clients' situations. It operates as what sociologists call a master status, a social status that is such a powerful label that it overshadows and contaminates all other identities an individual might have, such as mother or worker.[1] Consequently, addiction also serves as a way of understanding the social and economic aspects of women's lives. Drugs, crime, prostitution, unemployment, and abusive boyfriends are merely symptoms of the real problem deep inside women's selves. WTS staff members knew that their clients were often desperately poor, were caught in a dysfunctional legal system, and were likely to be survivors of sexual violence. The staff understood these experiences as the product of women's addiction to punishment. Their dependence had, in essence, led them to degrade themselves.

Yvonne, director of WTS's Legal Services Department, explained it to me this way: WTS clients needed "habilitation," not "rehabilitation," because they "don't even have a self" yet. Habilitation entails a complete resocialization, ultimately remaking the self because there is nothing there to rehabilitate. So for the staff, Sofia's focus on fixing things outside herself indicated addiction rather than normalization. The process of habilitation entailed transforming the women's selves in profound ways using therapeutic techniques. This ambitious project was backed by the criminal justice agencies that mandate women to WTS, giving the program enormous power over its clients. Yet WTS had lost power over Sofia. Prison no longer underpinned its authority. Consequently, staff members mobilized their last bits of leverage: her need for services and the program's power to stigmatize her as a criminal. In the end, Sofia decided to serve the rest of her time at WTS. She was there at graduation to celebrate overcoming her addiction to punishment.

In this chapter, I unpack how WTS understood addiction.[2] Where do these constructions come from? Why did they resonate with WTS staff members? How did they shape treatment? I argue that the program's construction of addiction distills the tropes and politics of the war on drugs. Criminal justice policies created penal rehab programs and thus shape WTS's goals, ideas, and therapeutic techniques, even as WTS framed itself as an alternative to harsh punishments. Scholars of the punitive turn have noted the system's important role in reproducing social inequality and argue that punishment has replaced other ways of governing poor marginal populations.[3] While confinement is one way of doing this, the state funds penal rehabs like WTS not only to control people but also to deal with the social and organizational crises produced by mass criminalization. Thus, governing through addiction combines penal control with the provision of welfare services. As a result, WTS's approach to addiction is not just about crime, it is also a strategy for managing social marginalization. Drawing on concerns about poor and black women's dependency, the addiction framework locates this problem in the self. While penal rehabs are a different sanction than imprisonment, I argue that WTS remains a punishment. Its therapeutic constructions carry with them carceral logics and techniques, which ultimately suspend citizenship just as traditional punishments do. In this chapter, I show that criminal sanctions possess a unique power to control and stigmatize. These essential features of punishment shape how institutions like WTS define addiction and organize treatment. Moreover, in the era of mass incarceration, the stigma of a criminal record is profoundly racialized and gendered.

CRIMINAL ADDICTS AND
GENDERED DEPENDENCY

Criminal justice institutions like the parole system have long treated employment as a signal of normalization. Some scholars of punishment interpret this as a sign that penal regimes function to support capitalism and racial hierarchies by producing docile laborers and disciplining subordinate classes.[4] Historically this focus on work applied particularly to men. In contrast, penal institutions attributed women's criminal behavior to their deviance from gender norms, so rehabilitation required training in domesticity. Throughout much of the twentieth century, women's prisons adopted familial and patriarchal regimes to embed inmates in the domestic environment that officials believed would foster supposedly normal womanhood.[5] Likewise, courts gave women lesser sentences if they were already ensconced in traditional familial controls, which meant that women who violated gender norms were punished more harshly.[6] Yet recent state efforts to normalize deviant women have focused on employment more than on domesticity, especially with the welfare reform that created Temporary Assistance to Needy Families. Spurred by panic over the dependency of poor and black women on the state, welfare reform signaled a shift in how the state valued women's private and public dependency. As a result, welfare now requires single mothers to work instead of requiring them to be full-time parents. At the same time that welfare became workfare, traditional ideas of correctional rehabilitation fell out of favor and were replaced by tough-on-crime policies. Most accounts of this punitive turn suggest that today's penal institutions simply warehouse people rather correcting them with work, religion, or therapy.[7] Even prisons for women seem to have dropped their long-standing commitment to domestic paternalism.[8] In penal rehabs, however, new ideas about reforming criminals are emerging. In these programs, addiction serves as the key framework for understanding and controlling crime and for envisioning what people need to be functioning citizens. In short, it is a mode of governance.

The term "habilitation" is not Yvonne's invention. It comes from an infamously harsh method of drug treatment called the therapeutic community (TC). TCs have roots in the radical self-help group Synanon, which was founded in 1958 by members of Alcoholics Anonymous (AA) who wanted a more demanding form of recovery.[9] TCs view addiction as a behavioral problem that results from having a poorly socialized immature self, with delusions of grandeur.[10] Jill McCorkel argues that habilitation is premised on the idea that addicts' selves are the cause of personal and social problems and thus need coercive resocialization.[11] TCs no longer exist only on the fringe. Because they are seen as tough, habilitation programs are the preferred treatment method in the criminal justice system, and government grants often require programs to be TCs. For example, New York State's Department of Corrections and Community Supervision does not use "rehabilitation" to describe its mission on its home page, instead describing itself as "responsible for the confinement and habilitation of approximately 53,000 individuals."[12] TCs are rarely found outside the penal state. This method is so pervasive that Yvonne uses the word "therapeutic" to mean punitive and militaristic. I initially found this quite confusing and assumed that she had misspoken. But Yvonne has the same training as most addiction counselors and a great deal of experience in treatment, having worked as an outpatient counselor for years before coming to WTS. Yvonne is also one of the most committed and eloquent proponents of WTS's take on addiction, and she was eventually promoted to director of the Residential Program. I realized the issue was mine: penal rehabs operate in such a distinct wing of the treatment field that they have their own terminology.

TCs fit so well into the penal system because their model of addiction dovetails with ideologies of the war on drugs that link drug use to poverty, moral decline, and racial minorities, especially African Americans. Studies of penal TCs find that the habilitation model focuses rehab on changing selves with harsh methods.[13] Addiction treatments have always used a mix of disciplinary, moral, and therapeutic techniques to shape the self.[14] However, today's penal rehabs are unusually intensive institutions. TCs rely on rigid hierarchy, confrontation, and humiliation to break down the false self, hold people accountable, and force behavioral change. Teresa Gowan and Sarah Whetstone argue that these "strong-arm rehabs" are "a primary site for the re-socialization and control of the poor," where quasi-medical ideas about addiction lead to the "biologization of poverty and race."[15] Kerwin Kaye's research on a TC program and a drug court show they defined addiction as a "drugs lifestyle" that resembles the "culture of poverty" thesis, which posits that nonwhite people are poor because they have a deviant culture rife with sexual promiscuity, welfare dependency, and an aversion to hard work.[16] In fact, Kaye found that TCs developed the term habilitation in the 1970s to refer to the needs of the poor and marginalized clients first entering TCs at that time. With the spread of penal rehabs, addiction discourse has moved concerns about the dependency of poor and marginalized groups from economic and moral frameworks into a framework about flawed selves.

Ideas about addiction and dependency also are deeply gendered. Although WTS does not call itself a TC, it draws on TC theories and techniques, mixing them with a hodgepodge of other methods to create a women-centered twist on habilitation. This makes WTS similar to most TCs, but with a less frequent use of confrontation and the addition of gender-responsive ideology. As in TCs, at WTS women spent most of their day in back-to-back group sessions. The social life of the residential setting does much of the therapeutic work, and women progress through hierarchical stages, gaining authority over lower-status clients. WTS uses distinctively TC lingo, too: the program is a "family" or "house," and fellow clients are "peers" or "sisters." Nevertheless, Yvonne is critical of using the standard TC method with women, although she did not see it as racialized. Echoing the critiques of many researchers, she told me that confrontational, militaristic treatment programs may work for men, but "you can't always do that with the women . . . because they come in with so much trauma. . . . They've been raped; they've been molested; they've been experiencing domestic violence; some of them have been tortured. And they just haven't been able to establish healthy relationships."[17] This method offended Yvonne, who explained that it replicates women's experiences with controlling and abusive men, which only foster drug use. Yvonne thought that men were tougher than women: "We probably can just cuss the men out all day," but women take that sort of thing personally. So women's treatment has to be "totally different." Thus, WTS bills itself as offering "comprehensive, client-centered, and humane" services so women can "reclaim their lives [and] reunite their families."

In blending TC-style habilitation with gendered recovery discourses, WTS still sees the self as the problem but views the problem as gendered. It argues that women's weak, traumatized selves are the root of addiction because women are dependent on outside sources of fulfillment and validation, which can include drugs, men, children, and even the street lifestyle. In self-help lingo, they are codependent. The subject of many best-selling books, codependency emerged from the twelve-step culture.[18] Unlike the original, male-dominated AA theory of addiction as an innate allergy to alcohol coupled with selfishness, codependency is a feminized problem linked to excessive neediness and caretaking.[19] In codependency discourse, what were once considered normal relations of dependence for women become pathological. However, in recovery texts, it is a woman's job to cure her codependency, and she does so by changing herself. She becomes autonomous by needing and expecting very little from other people or society.[20]

It may seem odd that this feminized wing of recovery culture would take root in the penal system. However, it was advocates for gender-responsive treatment for criminalized women who brought the codependency framework into punishment. Like staff members at WTS, these advocates linked codependency and trauma, pointing to the remarkably high rates of sexual abuse, rape, and domestic violence among women with substance abuse problems and those in the criminal justice system.[21] By 2005, even the Department of Justice had gotten on board, stating: "Gender-responsive treatment is essential to programs for females. These programs educate women and girls about self-esteem, self-sufficiency, and wellness and discuss topics such as codependent relationships and eating disorders."[22] When describing generic (that is, men's) treatment needs, the Department of Justice makes no mention of codependency. Notions of disordered dependency align with stereotypes about women, especially those who are poor and not white. In penal rehabs like WTS, addiction is a category rich with racial, class, and gender meanings—meanings that came from punitive discourses about crime and poverty.

The Person Is the Problem

One consequence of WTS's definition of addiction is that it deemphasizes drug use and crime. During staff meetings, the intake specialist quickly describes newly admitted women with a fairly standardized set of information: age, race, referral source, drug of choice, number of felonies, work experience, education, number of children, and whether she has cases with the city's child protective services (CPS) agency. But then comes the real introduction, in which staff members discuss the state of the client's self and what led her to such degradation, including her self-esteem, codependent family dynamics, and trauma from sexual victimization. Drugs and criminal offenses are rarely mentioned again. A client is thus defined more by whether she "intellectualizes everything," has "no relationship with herself," "uses men to validate herself," or "needs to work on her self-forgiveness." Staff members did not ignore drug use, but they saw it as merely a stepping-stone to other things. For example, Walter, a quiet black man who was a counselor in the Restabilization Program, brought up the case of Nadia, an Eastern European immigrant, who was an "ideal client" who followed all the rules. But Walter was concerned that she might relapse, which could be serious. Nadia had been hospitalized for alcohol poisoning twenty-five times in the past nine years. Walter worried that her drinking might be triggered by her boyfriend going out of town. Margaret, the social worker, mentioned that the boyfriend was also in recovery and wondered why he would be with someone like Nadia. Staff members were always skeptical of clients' relationships and spent a long time discussing Nadia's case. Then Marcus stepped in. He led the clinical team and was quite brilliant at developing explanations of clients' psyches. Marcus was charismatic but a bit domineering with both staff members and clients. One client even called him "a cock in the hen house."[23] Marcus said that Nadia needed to realize that drinking while her boyfriend is gone is not about him but about her. To figure out her triggers, Walter and Nadia should discuss her need for the relationship and consequent loneliness, the real source of her drinking.

WTS's fixation on the self rather than drug use or following rules can be seen in the kinds of infractions that earned clients an unsuccessful discharge from the program. This was the most serious sanction WTS had. Such women were referred back to court or to parole, which would either send them to prison or to a different, often more restrictive, facility. During my fieldwork at WTS, I never saw a woman be discharged for relapsing. On the other hand, if a woman seemed uninterested in intensive therapeutic work on the self, she was in trouble. Ella, a sensitive black woman near forty, relapsed four months into her time in the Residential Program. Out a pass, Ella had a difficult meeting with her estranged daughter. After that, Ella absconded, took crack cocaine, and showed up at a court date a few days later. WTS readmitted her, and I saw her looking unusually disheveled in parenting class. Clearly in despair but willing to share her problems, Ella explained to the class that her daughter had said hurtful things to her, so she had gone back to doing what she did well: using. Then Ella tearfully concluded that she was not ready to see her daughter again, whom she described as "more of a harm than a good."

Ella's relapse provoked a debate at that week's staff meeting. Some counselors worried that by readmitting her they had not followed the rules. Ella had already been on a forty-five-day "contract," which is the terminology WTS uses for its punishments. Contracts usually involve reduced privileges, writing long essays about your issues, and performing extra chores. Moreover, the staff had been about to review Ella's contract to consider extending it and making it more severe. Contracts typically stipulate that the client will be discharged if she fails to abide by the rules, which of course include no drug use. Linda, a Latina counselor who had good relations with the clients, said that many of them were mad that Ella had been allowed to return to the program because she continued to act "superior" despite relapsing. Even with these concerns, Ella stayed. However, she was demoted back to the beginning orientation level. A similar thing happened when Roxanne relapsed on a pass and was transferred to the more restrictive Residential Program.

After a discussion about how relapsing was part of the recovery process, the staff rescinded a discharge for Denise, a black woman in her twenties who had tested positive on a random urinalysis. They brought Denise into their meeting to tell her the good news. Rachel, a senior counselor and a black woman in her forties, then scolded Denise for recently "deviating on a pass" outside the facility to buy breakfast. Denise was allowed to go only to a nearby coffee cart, but she had gone instead to a store that was a few feet away. When clients leave on a pass, they are usually "escorted" by a higher-ranking client who is rewarded for informing staff of any "deviations." Denise's escort reported her for going to the store. Denise tried to defend herself, saying she didn't drink coffee and so had gone to the store to get a soda. Rachel shot her down, asking "Do you know why we expect that?" Rachel answered herself: the staff members were upset because Denise had disobeyed instructions. Denise tried again to explain herself. Rachel interrupted to impress on her that allowing her to stay after relapsing meant that she would really have to follow the rules and listen to her escort. When she is told to go get coffee and a bagel, that is what she should get. Denise nodded and thanked them for letting her back in. After she was gone Marcus told Rachel, "I am on the client's side on this one." He thought that rules should mean something and said he didn't drink coffee either. Rachel countered that she was trying to teach Denise to understand rules and to negotiate the situation without blowing off her escort. Despite disagreeing about Denise's latest infraction, the staff had agreed about how to handle her relapse.

While relapse was part of what staff called "the process," one woman was forcibly discharged for a suspected sexual relationship with another client. Another woman who secretly stopped taking her bipolar medication was referred back to court for being noncompliant. A third was referred back to the parole system after being arrested for pickpocketing, and according to Walter was headed to "do time." Jay, WTS's court liaison, commented that this client had never been interested in treatment; she just wanted help with her legal cases. The woman suspected of having a sexual relationship had been found with another client in the dark, in one of WTS's common rooms. She claimed she was there to get a videotape but was not holding one. This incident caused a small scandal among the counselors, who assumed she was lying. Marcus said he had previously spoken to her about not getting into relationships during treatment. The staff discharged her because they concluded she was not committed. Yet they determined this not from her lying, which they reported many clients doing; it was the mere fact of the relationship that signaled she was unwilling to work on the self. She broke one of WTS's "cardinal rules," "no sexually acting out." Another cardinal rule was "no drugs."[24] Yet in reality one was taken more seriously than the other.

When the staff met to discuss clients, they had to define what was wrong with these women. Clients at WTS had many concerns and problems, so the staff had to do interpretive work to determine which of these needs were their job. Rehabs and penal institutions have used various logics to define women's needs. At WTS, the staff consistently used penal definitions of addiction to frame women's problems as problems of the self, which had solely therapeutic solutions. This approach required a particularly intimate kind of surveillance. Counselors pooled information about clients' pasts, family dynamics, victimization, psychiatric diagnoses, self-presentation, and emotional states. This was why the meetings were so long. As a result, the most common reason I saw counselors get in trouble was for not communicating all they knew about clients. When things went wrong, Marcus invariably berated his staff with the refrain, "We are a *treatment* facility!" For WTS, transforming selves was the essence of treatment.

From Welfare to Work on the Self

WTS's definition of addiction blotted out the social and economic forces that shaped women's lives, thus making it hard for staff members to figure out what place its welfare services should have in treatment. As a result, they really struggled with clients who were uninterested in therapeutic work on the self. During one meeting, Margaret turned to her colleagues for advice on what to do with Charlene. A white woman and the only social worker on staff, Margaret had significant influence on the clinical team. She sounded exasperated when she explained that Charlene was "resistant to all services." Charlene "had questions" about why she was in this type of program. She was interested only in what Margaret called "concrete services"—specifically, help finding housing and managing her chronic health problems. So Charlene "avoids anything regarding counseling" and "focuses on not being here." Carl, a young African American vocational counselor, agreed. Charlene had told him that she was "not really here." Since WTS's services did not focus on what she thought she needed, Charlene hoped to get her mandated stay shortened to ninety days. Her case provoked a long, uneasy discussion.

The staff members in the room immediately agreed that Charlene's interest in "concrete services" and lack of interest in working on her self subverted the proper focus of treatment. Various staff members participated in building this interpretation by sharing stories of what Charlene had said or done that indicated a disordered self. For instance, she had been diagnosed as being bipolar, but she did not want to take medication. One counselor mentioned that Charlene frequently used her health issues to get time on bed rest, rather than going to the group sessions where clients spent most of their time. Another noted that Charlene's use of bed rest sparked other clients' resentment. "The community" accused Charlene of "buying time"—that is, going through the program simply to get out of a prison sentence. Someone then brought up Charlene's complaint about WTS's medical services, noting that she had contacted another agency serving criminalized women to look for assistance, which the staff found suspicious. Margaret suggested that the counseling, legal, intake, and housing departments "case conference" Charlene. Case conferences are one of WTS's more serious disciplinary measures, in which multiple staff members confront a client about her poor progress.

Then Marcus wondered out loud why they were so invested in getting Charlene to stay. I too thought that staff members seemed desperate to prove Charlene wrong. This self-analysis was a common practice at meetings, often initiated by Marcus. What if she *is* a bad fit for WTS, he asked, playing devil's advocate. In an unusual move, the staff briefly considered the possibility that Charlene actually did not have a drug problem—she did not have an extensive history of drug use. But this idea did not get very far. The counselors returned to the notion that Charlene displayed deeper problems. Her focus on "concrete services" was manipulation. She had tried to "split the staff" in two by convincing some that she was a bad fit. In addition, some staff members claimed that she had serious "trust issues" and felt the need to please other people, which were signs of codependency. Regardless of her drug use, these behaviors indicated that she was an addict and needed WTS's treatment. Margaret decided that Charlene "used" her illnesses to "decompensate." In other words, her requests for medical accommodations and housing services were signs that she was falling apart. I was typing up official notes of the meeting, and they instructed me to write that WTS would reassess Charlene's fit with "this modality" of treatment. But Margaret also resolved to go ahead with the disciplinary "case conference." Two weeks later, WTS denied Charlene a "level movement," which is a promotion in status that indicates success in one stage of treatment. She absconded the following week. It is likely that a warrant was then issued for her arrest.

Charlene troubled the WTS counselors with her lack of interest in therapeutic self-improvement. Margaret described Charlene's emphasis on housing and health care as being "resistant to all services," momentarily forgetting that these other services are also part of WTS. By the end of the conversation, Charlene's lack of interest in therapy had become a sign that she needed therapy. This is a classic dynamic in institutions of social control. Once an individual is labeled with a deviant identity, his or her behavior is inevitably interpreted in light of that label.[25] Pooling information about clients' issues aided control as well as diagnosis. The staff sought to ensure that women were not able to manipulate the program through presenting a false self. They were perpetually concerned that clients were using the program for its nontherapeutic services. Penal institutions for women have a long history of constructing inmates as manipulative, but WTS's narrative of addiction included the racial baggage of the dependent welfare queen, who bilks the state out of money.[26] However, staff members never really thought clients were after money per se. One woman was suspected of trying to be diagnosed with mental illness to get disability benefits. Another woman was suspected of being such a skilled manipulator that that she was able to delude several psychiatrists into thinking she did not have a mental illness. What tied these instances together was that they revealed women's lack of self-knowledge and addictive traits. In the codependency framework, what Nancy Fraser and Linda Gordon call the "moral/psychological register" of dependency subsumes what was previously seen as economic or social dependence.[27] As a result, WTS problematizes women who rely on anything outside themselves. These women did not need services; they needed to work on their selves.

Staff members used clients' interest in services to gain therapeutic access to their inner selves. For instance, clients could leave the facility to go to educational programs or find a job only if they had good performance in the therapeutic aspects of program. Kate was just about to graduate and showed outward signs of success. She worked and was in training to be an administrative assistant. Consequently, the drug court released her from its mandate. Carl, her vocational counselor, said that she was eager to leave and had already found a realtor to help her find an apartment. Another counselor, Lucy, reported that Kate's explanation for her recent flurry of activity was that she was "at her best" when she was productive. But Lucy thought Kate was in trouble because she still presented with the "same behaviors" as when she arrived and was "not working on internal issues." This was evident when Kate made "impulse purchases," was "cocky," "manipulate[d]," and gave money away to "feel superior." As the discussion continued, staff members characterized Kate's focus on work as merely a desire for validation. Lucy decided that Kate should follow up with WTS's after-care program. However, Kate had declined to do so, claiming that she did not need it.

This example of her "cockiness" was the final straw for Marcus. He stood up and yelled at his staff. Kate's priorities revealed the failure of WTS's treatment. Looking pointedly at Carl, Marcus claimed that Kate had the "same issues going out" as she did coming in because WTS let her go to work too early. Marcus said that Kate should not have been permitted to work at a job if she wasn't working on "treatment." She couldn't use vocational services and "not do treatment!" Marcus noted that they would find other clients like this. Then he listed several other women while counting on his fingers, saying "they are not even my clients; I just see them and know they are like this." He declared Kate a waste of time. She was never really committed, Marcus decided. So WTS should have referred her back to the court and taken someone else instead. But Carl disagreed. He argued that work was important and that lots of clients were not ready to deal with their issues. Marcus responded that WTS's funders and the state licensing agency would see reports of clients leaving with the same issues and wonder what on earth WTS was doing—implying that staff members' jobs and the program itself were on the line.

After discussing Kate, the staff turned back to Sofia. She had stayed, but Karen was still worried about her. Sofia had not gotten the necessary things ready for being out on her own. She had "problems budgeting" and spent too much on grooming and her children. This, Karen thought, was because she was too focused on studying for a medical assistant's license and not focused enough on herself. In fact, Sofia was again trying to leave because WTS was too "chaotic" for her to study. Karen asked her colleagues how Sofia would manage being a single parent, working, and going to school. Sofia was "OCD" (had obsessive-compulsive disorder) and "taking on too much." To succeed at

WTS, Sofia had to work on her self rather than toward a career if she wanted to be ready for reentering society. So, Karen announced, she would to talk to Sofia's parole officer. In a notable flip-flop from his views about Kate's case, Marcus defended Sofia's focus on school. To support the position that she was "decompensating," Karen pointed to Sofia's additional emotional problems: she was obsessed with her daughter's having premarital sex and making the same mistakes that she had made. After supporting Sofia's focus on school, Marcus changed his tune when he heard that she was not keeping up with her psychiatric medications. The staff was regularly frustrated by having to deal with what are known as mentally ill chemically addicted (MICA), or dual-diagnosis, clients. While some programs specialize in this population, WTS did not. Yet it had many clients with psychiatric diagnoses, and it was often difficult for referral agencies and WTS staff members to tell when clients needed a more specialized program. When discussing Sofia, Marcus became increasingly frustrated and emphasized that "we are not a MICA facility!" Patricia added that another client had recently been sent back to WTS from a job placement program with the instruction that she should be in a "MICA home." This was too much for Marcus, who exclaimed, "We are a treatment facility!" The divided staff agreed to do a "case conference" with Sofia.

As the staff assessed Kate, Charlene, and Sofia, they disregarded these women's own assessment of their needs and instead viewed them according to WTS's definition of addiction. MICA clients were especially difficult because they infringed on WTS's understanding of the problem and undermined the feasibility of its solutions. Yet plenty of women at WTS were on psychiatric drugs. Only when psychiatric issues seemed to overshadow issues of the self did women become candidates for the MICA label and ejection from WTS. While WTS emphasized women's psychologies, these were neither typical mental health diagnoses nor traditional legal measures of normalization. They were issues distinct to the addiction framework used in penal rehabs. For instance, Kate was dependent on the validation of work, rather than working to find self-validation through greater self-knowledge and self-esteem. While Carl defended Kate's ability to work for pay while working on her self, Lucy and Marcus thought the self had to come first. Moreover, Marcus observed that transforming selves was what the state expected the program to do. The staff defined women's needs as internal rather than social. Consequently, access to welfare services, and thus to social citizenship, was contingent on "working on the self." In short, WTS saw women like Kate and Sofia as not empowered enough for freedom.

WTS staff members are quite proud of the program's gender-sensitive approach and think it challenges the racism and sexism of the criminal justice system. The program's website features statistics about the racial, class, and gender disadvantages facing women in prison, and the executive director advocates publicly for alternatives to incarceration. At one graduation, she movingly argued that WTS women are "worth celebrating and fighting for." Moreover, the state tasks WTS with managing complex social problems. In this context, women's "addiction to pain and punishment" serves as a way of understanding how these forms of oppression operate. Karen was right to worry about whether Sofia could handle work, school, and being a single mother. "Having it all" is hard for any woman, let alone one who is poor and has the burden of a felony conviction, which substantially hurts an individual's chance at getting a job.[28] So when Karen argued for the importance of finding validation in the self, she was trying arm Sofia for a world where she could, in fact, expect very little from the state or the labor market. I found that WTS staff members were regularly skeptical that their clients would find meaningful work or supportive relationships. In less sympathetic moments, they claimed women needed "reality therapy." I asked Margaret how, as a counselor, she dealt with the role of poverty and racial inequality in her clients' lives. She acknowledged that these factors were hugely important, but she did not bring them up with clients because she worried it would make them feel hopeless. Focusing on the self, Margaret implied, would create feelings of possibility. Therapeutic governance through personal "recovery" appealed to the staff because it promised self-esteem in the face of huge obstacles. Staffers knew they could do little to change the larger structures that disadvantaged WTS clients, so they opted for changing the women instead.[29] However, by locating the problem in the self, the addiction framework worked against WTS's ostensible goals. It consistently individualized women's problems, blamed them for their own victimization and disadvantage, and justified excluding them from meaningful citizenship.

PUNISHMENT OUTSIDE THE PRISON

WTS's approach drew on therapeutic discourses, but it depended on the organization's power to punish. In *Discipline and Punish*, Michel Foucault famously argued that many modern, supposedly enlightened institutions like schools and mental hospitals deploy the same practices of discipline, surveillance, and normalization used in prisons.[30] This insight revealed that such institutions share an insidious kind of power: they attempt to change the soul. Foucault's influential idea produced a great deal of scholarship showing that therapeutic techniques are ubiquitous tools for governing conduct and encouraging self-regulation. Moreover, through these strategies, power acts on people in the name of freeing them.[31] I went into my research with this argument about the pervasiveness of disciplinary control in mind. Indeed, WTS and Gladstone Lodge share many such practices. The influence of self-help culture on WTS reveals that penal institutions are shaped by larger trends in governance. However, for all the counselors' emphasis on the psyche, confession, and self-management, I found that WTS remained irreducibly a punishment. This hinged on two features of WTS: its powers to control and to stigmatize. During my fieldwork there, I was often impressed with the organization's critiques of incarceration and its lofty aim of empowering women. Yet WTS could not escape the coercive and stigmatizing aspects of punishment. In fact, its methods required them. WTS did not, in the end, deploy the same mode of governance as Gladstone Lodge. To understand this, I turned to other theories of punishment that argue it has a unique ability to label individuals as stigmatized others.[32] In this perspective, punishment has a distinctive cultural role: producing meanings that mark social boundaries. Through its construction of addiction and its methods of treatment, WTS stigmatized and coerced women, depriving them of full citizenship. And it depended on the state's power to punish to carry out this task.

The Stigma of a Criminal Label

Parole mandated Leena to WTS after a positive drug test. When I arrived at the legal services office, she was on her way to the facility from her mother's house, and staff members were already talking about her. Ayana, a young black woman who was the intake specialist, told me that Leena had a "reputation." Because of this Ayana predicted that Leena would be trouble. Ayana explained that Leena had been in treatment before, became a counselor, and eventually worked her way up to a director's position. Ayana also said that Leena had lied to her employers about having a master's degree. What is more, she was currently in school and had made special arrangements to leave WTS on two days during her first week so she could take her final exams. Clients are generally not permitted to leave for a month. Ayana's irritation reflected a sense that Leena had asked for a reward before she earned one. So Leena's efforts to ensure that she could finish her semester only worsened her "reputation," making her seem arrogant, entitled, and fussy. Ayana explained what I should expect: Leena would "talk herself up" and start "bragging" right away about how educated she is.

When Leena arrived in the reception area, Yvonne burst into the office laughing and said that Leena looked like she was going to a job interview. Ayana peeked out the door to the main hallway and snickered with Yvonne at Leena's hair and clothing. To compose herself, Ayana looked at me, announced that she would "put on my happy face," and took a deep breath before going out to get Leena. I sat in the corner of the crowded office and watched the intake process, wondering if Leena would live up to the hype. She was African American and probably in her early thirties. She was dressed nicely in slacks, as if for an office job, and her hair was curled and neat. I thought she seemed demure rather than arrogant. Leena and I sat in awkward silence while Ayana went over paperwork. Eventually Leena broke the silence to ask a few questions about WTS's program and the pass to take her exams. Ayana conducted the intake screening, inquiring about Leena's family history, drug use, sexual past, legal situation, mental health, medical history, education, and more. Leena was cooperative throughout. Afterward, she asked if she could call her mother to say that she had arrived safely. Ayana allowed her to make the call on the office phone, instead of the pay phone clients typically had to use.

Ayana mentioned that Leena was mandated to WTS for six months, and Leena looked shocked. There must be a misunderstanding, she said—it should be three months. Skeptical, Ayana called Leena's parole officer to straighten it out. He left it up to WTS. It never seemed important to him or Ayana what the original mandate was. But it mattered to Leena. Seeming more than a little desperate at the idea of serving six months, Leena explained that she had only used cocaine twice and had been caught both times. She had learned her lesson, she declared, so she should get only three months. Ayana's expression was deadpan. I could not tell if she believed this story. While Leena made her case, Ayana meticulously searched her luggage for contraband, unrolling her neatly packed clothes and opening bottles of toiletries and makeup bags. Anxiously Leena then asked a series of questions to make sure she could get to her exams. Some of them were oral exams given by several professors, so she could not reschedule them, she emphasized. Leena wanted to know how this special pass would work, how long it lasted, and if she was sure to get it. She expressed concern about whether she would have time to study in the next few days. Leena succeeded only in exasperating Ayana, who pointedly noted that WTS was making a generous exception by giving her that pass. Leena did not look reassured.

After the intake interview, Patricia came in to get Leena for a ritual that WTS calls "induction." In her typically firm fashion, Patricia explained that Leena had to take a shower with delousing soap while staff members watched. Leena sighed, looked annoyed, and said, "I didn't know [this] was like [Bayard]," a state prison where she had served time. Leena went on to explain that her hair was in "a press 'n' curl do," which would lose all its styling if it got wet. Increasingly alarmed, she clarified that this could not happen because she needed to look presentable for her oral exams. She asked if she could be put "in isolation" until after the exams to preserve her hairstyle. Patricia laughed condescendingly at the idea and said, "This is not prison; there is no isolation." Leena then asked if she could go to a salon to redo her hair after the induction. No. Finally, one staff member suggested they find another client with the equipment and skills to do a press 'n' curl. Eventually they found Denise, who even knew Leena from prison.

As Leena gathered her things to head off to the induction, she reiterated that she had only done cocaine twice and should have to stay for only three months. But she left without knowing how long she would stay. Leena's claim struck me as implausible, and I figured the staff would not believe her. After she had left, I asked Ayana if she often heard that kind of thing. Ayana, to my surprise, seemed willing to believe her. Puzzled, I asked Ayana why parole would send someone who was not an addict to treatment. Ayana was not bothered by this at all. She shrugged and explained that Leena's parole officer thought "she needed structure." I did not say this out loud, but I immediately thought that many people "need structure" but are not punished for that. Indeed, I was then struggling with time management in graduate school. I "needed structure," too. But because of the intertwining of the criminal justice system with racial and class inequality, Leena ended up getting deloused, and I ended up researching her.

WTS's induction serves as what sociologists call a "degradation ceremony." Harold Garfinkel developed this term to describe the rituals used by courts and penal institutions to transform an offender's identity into one with a lower status.[33] In his study of total institutions, Erving Goffman argued that these sorts of rituals contribute to a "mortification of the self" that strips inmates of their past normal identity and its markers.[34] These aspects of punishment may have practical goals such as preventing infestation, but they also communicate moral condemnation and reinforce the higher status of the punishers. After her induction, Leena would find herself in therapeutic groups with names like "Gettin' Honest," "Reclaiming Lives," and "Encounters with Self." Although Patricia told her WTS was "not prison," Leena immediately recognized the similarity between the two. WTS is an alternative sanction operating in the community, but it is still administering punishment—which requires stigma and coercion. This went beyond induction. Yvonne and Ayana stigmatized Leena as a criminal by depicting her as an addict who was manipulative, cocky, and unable to manage herself. The addict label served to increase WTS's power to punish Leena when the parole officer mandated her to receive treatment for needing structure and then left it up to WTS to decide how long the treatment should be.

WTS officially aspires to help women meet their educational and vocational goals; its staff members even taught clients how to dress for job interviews. Leena would seem to be ahead of the curve, a relatively easy case. However, Leena's professional appearance and education were not well received. Many WTS clients had been in treatment before, but few had worked in treatment centers, let alone as managers. In the face of a possible challenge to the staff's authority, Ayana and Yvonne worked to reassert Leena's lower status by mocking her ambition and discounting her accomplishments. Yet staff members had much in common with their clients. Quite a few counselors were former addicts and had likely had run-ins with the law; and many came from socioeconomic backgrounds similar to those of the clients.[35] Marcus initially defended Sofia's focus on schooling because she (unlike Kate) was willing to participate in therapeutic aspects of WTS. On top of that, Marcus was going to college while working full-time at WTS, a situation that was clearly very stressful. But there were limits to staff members' willingness to identify with clients, because their clients were so stigmatized. Counselors often scoffed at clients' vocational goals, especially if they wanted to become addiction counselors. Case review meetings were regularly derailed by gossipy discussions about why clients' romantic partners would be interested in them or how much food they ate. Similar backgrounds did provide staff members with opportunities for identifying with clients, but they also required staffers to do work to assert their higher status and ensure their legitimacy. What is more, staff members did not have many status resources to draw on. Substance abuse counseling is a paraprofessional field, and WTS is in a feminized, low-paying, privatized branch of the penal system. Staffers do not have the badges, weapons, or job benefits that state correctional employees get. Theirs was not an easy position, and that fact accentuated the importance of stigma.

Through its definition of addiction, WTS imparts a stigma that is distinctly based on race, gender, and class. As poor and (mostly) nonwhite women who have used drugs, WTS clients are among the most vilified groups in the country. Monstrous crack mothers and their pathological families were centerpieces of the war on drugs. When WTS framed addiction as a totalizing disorder located in an unsocialized self, it continued to mark its clients with this stigma. As later chapters show, addiction did not impart the same stigma at Gladstone Lodge. WTS's therapeutic take on addiction did not draw directly on criminal categories or overt moral language. In fact, it was trying to counter these approaches. However, the TC-based narrative of addiction was intertwined with racialized ideas about crime. This became clear when women were depicted as manipulative welfare queens and pathologically dependent. The very concept of addiction undermines the existence of agency and willpower, but at WTS this dependency encompassed all of the self and one's social relationships. Such constructions of the will have a racial history. The legal scholar Patricia Williams writes: "One of the things passed on from slavery, which continues in the oppression of people of color, is the belief structure rooted in a concept of black (or brown or red) antiwill, the antithetical embodiment of pure will. We live in a society where the closest equivalent of nobility is the display of unremittingly controlled willfulness. To be perceived as unremittingly without will is to be imbued with an almost lethal trait."[36]

By making work on the self come first, WTS treated women as so dysfunctional that they could not yet participate in society. Thus it suspended
women's citizenship just as traditional punishments do. Through the notion
that its clients are addicted to punishment, WTS legitimated the need for
coercive penal control of their entire lives.

Punishment and Control

Another feature of WTS that made it a punishment was its enormous
power to control its clients. WTS's intensive therapeutic project depended on
practices of coercion that were underpinned by the state's power to punish.
The penal state gave WTS important resources not found in other kinds of
rehab programs: time, services, and a legal mandate. A number of practices
flowed from this coercive power. For example, it enabled WTS to engage clients in deep work. Because the clients stayed at WTS for many months, the
program could tackle the huge terrain of the self and sequester women from
their lives. Even groups that were ostensibly didactic, such as parenting class,
emphasized feelings of shame, traumatic experiences, and family conflicts.
Moreover, the staff was able to use the program's material and legal services
as leverage to get clients to buy into the therapeutic project. Thus, WTS also
used the clients' poverty and marginality to its advantage. Women sometimes
resisted this power, as when Ella and Charlene absconded, but WTS was able
to use the threat of incarceration or the loss of a client's children to press for
compliance. Counselors deeply valued the legal mandate, saying that it was
important to making treatment work. At the same time, WTS's practices and
therapeutic language worked to conceal the coercive power of the program,
including from the staff members themselves. The rhetoric of contracts, which
clients signed like a legal agreement, produced a fiction of voluntariness.
However, clients described this condition as "being on a contract," depicting
it as coercive rather than mutual.

The cases of Kate, Sofia, and Charlene also show that WTS gave women
little autonomy to decide their own fates. This was a common theme. As
women were about to complete the program, WTS needed to find them
housing. Because of their concerns about dependency, counselors always tried
to keep women from moving in with their families or partners. However,
there are limited housing options available to women who are poor and have
criminal records. So WTS pushed clients to live in single-room-occupancy
facilities (SROs) or halfway houses, because they considered such places to
be more independent, even though they entailed greater supervision. Tracie,
a mellow black counselor, ran a group to help women apply for housing
assistance. Tracie began by assuming that everyone would go into a SRO. She
explained all the details about the paperwork and waiting periods. Desiree, a

poised black client, raised her hand and said that she had gotten information about an SRO and wanted to know if it was okay to pursue this herself. Tracie said that Desiree still had to come to her and submit the paperwork. Desiree looked angry and asked, "So we can't do our own footwork?" Tracie insisted that Desiree go through her, and Desiree sat back with a look that suggested she was not surprised.

Next Shavon raised her hand and, sounding distressed, said that she had a drug felony so she was not eligible for Section 8 (a federal housing subsidy program). But she needed to have housing to get custody of her kids, and she would not get her kids back from foster care if she was living in a SRO. Tracie suggested that she move into a SRO, work, and save money for an apartment: "Be patient." Shavon looked disappointed. Tracie then went on about one SRO that was "real nice." It was a "structured living environment. . . . A lot of people think it's a program. It's not a program." As I listened to the women's questions and Tracie's answers, it sounded more and more like a program to me: no visitors were allowed, there was a curfew, each resident had a case worker and was expected to go to Narcotics Anonymous meetings, and residents' urine was tested for drugs each week. Tracie said that while it was good to want "to move on with your life," it is still important to have structure. Sensing that this was not convincing, Tracie then described a mother-child program with nice apartments. Shavon asked if residents could "live there forever." No, Tracie acknowledged; it was "transitional housing" where residents were regularly drug tested. Shavon made a noise that indicated disapproval. Tracie retorted, "but if you clean, you shouldn't mind [submitting] your urine every day." Annoyed, Shavon responded, "but I want to be like a normal person and not always have to be giving my urine to someone." Tracie followed by reiterating her advice to move into an SRO and save money.

Shavon did not see this kind of surveillance as normal for an independent person. Nor would living in an SRO allow her to reunite with her children. Desiree wanted to arrange her housing herself but had to go through WTS. Both women asserted their own definitions of what it means to be free of dependency and able to act on one's own behalf. But WTS advocated an odd sort of individualism, one that required a lot of external control. During this group, women discussed the requirements of CPS, asked questions about various housing subsidy programs, and tried to remember all the agencies where they had case workers. Through this process they tried to convince Tracie about the material supports and legal rights they would need to be a "normal person." However, WTS's preference for "independent living" in SROs and the limited housing assistance for mothers with drug convictions left Tracie with few "normal" options to offer. Tracie's conflicts with Shavon and Desiree reveal the contradictions that arise from a therapeutic definition of autonomy.

Not surprisingly, these conflicts emerged around issues of women's economic and social needs, which the addiction framework failed to grasp.

WTS draws on treatment techniques from TCs that merge therapy with punishment and depend on WTS's coercive power as well as the clients' degraded status. These techniques include having to do punitive chores and write essays about one's issues, confrontations, and—according to something I heard from a volunteer but did not see myself—making women wear shaming signs hung around their neck saying things like "thief" and "liar." In fact, Yvonne told me that when she first started working at WTS she was shocked at how staff members would yell at clients. She eventually got used to it. Yvonne explained WTS's difference from TCs this way: "We also use a confrontation setting, but we call it care and concern." She noted there is an "an art" to confrontation, and women must walk away knowing that the program cares about them. Because WTS did not use confrontational encounter groups very often, I was never able to observe the harshest version, in which a woman is singled out while the other clients hurl criticisms at her, but such confrontations did happen on occasion, especially when the counselors felt that the resident population was "wild" and "unbalanced."

If staff members thought things were really bad, WTS would "close the house" for several days to force clients to work on their selves even more intensively. When the house is closed, clients may not leave the facility and all family visits and passes are rescinded. Speaking outside of group sessions is banned. When I arrived one day when the house was closed, an exhausted client told me, "we be grouping like sixteen to eighteen hours a day!" My shocked face made her laugh and nod. The staff had told her this was done in all treatment programs, but she saw it as "punishment." Margaret told me that one multiday speaking ban was because clients were "bickering and being loud." This sounds minor, but she sounded very stern and angry to convey how serious this was. During that day's case review meeting, a frustrated Marcus proclaimed that the clients were "all immature" and "99 percent have poor impulse control." In parenting class that evening, with the speaking ban still in place, the clients watched videos on how to speak to children with respect. In one video, a scene depicted a mother doing the wrong thing when she yelled at a resistant boy and gave him ultimatums. Another scene showed her doing the right thing, giving the boy choices—something the women at WTS did not often have.

However, there are limits to WTS's authority, especially because it is located in the community and does not have full custodial control of its clients. When women relapsed, it was almost always outside the facility, and in several cases they were on WTS-granted passes. I heard of many contracts for women who stayed out too long on a pass or went somewhere they were not permitted to go. These infractions were usually more minor than getting high. For example, one pair of women was put on a contract for getting their nails done after work, when they were expected to return directly to WTS. Clients did use passes as sites for resistance. I found that they enjoyed these little trips away from the facility and used them to gain feelings of independence and normalcy. During a smoking break, one woman described going to visit her parole officer once a month. "It's beautiful," she said with such seriousness and meaning that I initially thought she must be joking. But she continued, "I go alone." For her, WTS was so controlling that she experienced going to the parole office by herself as liberating. Community-based correctional facilities like WTS are supposed to work as reintegrating institutions, rebuilding individuals' connections to family and society. Yet this proximity to the outside poses real challenges for WTS. Demanding that clients focus on their selves was one way WTS tried to deal with this tension. But not all community correctional facilities have developed an emphasis on the self, so the proximity of the outside world cannot itself explain WTS's approach. It was the program's construction of the problem that rendered women as a particular kind of criminal, an addicted one unfit for even the most basic freedoms.

"You Are Your Sister's Keeper": Surveillance and Privacy

In addition to curtailing women's ability to control their own lives, WTS used surveillance techniques that depended on its power to punish. All residential programs use a group living environment to change people, but TCs particularly emphasize mutual surveillance and hierarchal relations among clients. In the prison-based TC that McCorkel studied, staff members posted large pictures of blue eyes on the wall with the menacing phrase "the eyes are always watching you."[37] At WTS, the practice of escorting was one example, but peer surveillance was deeply engrained throughout the therapeutic process. As a result, women had no space outside of treatment, and everything they did was fodder for discipline. Once a week, WTS's two inpatient programs, Residential and Restabilization, gather for a meeting called "House Matters," at which clients hear announcements and discuss house business. House meetings are structured as ritualized public confessions. Women air their feelings, confess deviations, and admonish fellow clients in what is called a "pull up." The clients sit in a large circle, while most staff members stand crowded together at the doorway, watching. At one house meeting, a client complained about having "no me time"—a desire I thought the program would support, given its goal of work on the self. But Patricia, who had been sitting in the circle with clients, intervened to chastise the woman: "It doesn't take time away from yourself to reach out to another human being!" She told the woman she needed "to live life on life's terms." Many clients nodded in agreement. Then Patricia brought up Roxanne's recent relapse, claiming that they should have seen it coming and intervened: "[Roxanne] dying and all of you not noticing!" Patricia told them, "You are your sister's keeper." In this way, house meetings incorporated peer and staff surveillance with therapeutic aims and the mundane concerns of living together. As a result, WTS often succeeded in recruiting clients into governing one another, and the atmosphere at the meetings was typically contentious.

One day, I arrived for the meeting when the house was closed. The client designated to run the meeting asked if there were any contracts, which clients must confess to the group. Whitney stood up, gave her name, and said that she was on a forty-five-day extended contract, but no one could understand her mumbled explanation. After a pause another client stood up and said that she was on a "last-chance contract for acting out and being disrespectful." She then asked the assembled clients to give her a "pull up" if they saw her reverting to her old behavior. Following the required ritual sequence, she asked, "Can I get that?" The clients said "yes" in unison. Then Marcus asked if everyone had understood Whitney. The other clients said no. So Whitney stood up again and said she was on a contract for going to the store without permission. Marcus asked her to specify why the contract had been extended, and she said because she had drunk caffeinated coffee during the week. But Whitney did not make the ritualized request "can I get help with that?" One counselor told her to say it "or you will be out." Whitney still refused, and then many clients piped up, begging her to say it. After this tense moment, a third woman got up to announce that she was on a contract for disrespecting her peers and asked for help with that. The group responded loudly, "yes!"

The meeting moved on to "pull ups," where the women debated who had been helping with the kitchen work and if the division of the chores was fair. Because of the requirement that clients perform chores, these kinds of conflicts were common at both WTS and Gladstone Lodge. However, at the Lodge chores were systematically rotated and never used as a punishment. Consequently, chores and cleanliness were more divisive at WTS, and women often used them against each other. Zorida prefaced her complaint with "we're all grown women here" and said that she had walked into the bathroom and stepped on urine that had been all over the floor. Several women in the meeting looked shocked and disgusted. Zorida reiterated: "we are grown" and so "you should get that yourselves." Finally Tiffany, who was quite young and new to treatment, stood up and complained rather incoherently that she didn't like "the house" holding her problems with her boyfriend against her. Trudy, the house manager and a much-loved motherly woman, shook her head with dismay as Tiffany spoke. These were precisely the kind of issues that were part of treatment. Some clients smirked at Tiffany's mistake and shared knowing glances. After Tiffany sat down, her counselor prompted her to get back up and apologize to the house for getting something out of the vending machine while she was being escorted out of the facility. Tiffany stood up and said defensively that she didn't know she wasn't supposed to do that. Her actions were unusual. It was not typical for women to make excuses for their relationships and desires—this was not the purpose of the public confession.

The meeting moved on to "good feelings." During this section, Desiree stood up to tell us excitedly that her sister, whom she hadn't seen in nineteen years, had found her and called WTS. Desiree recounted that her sister was worried about her and would come get her when she got out and take her "home." Desiree's voice cracked with emotion as she said "home." This news was received with eager applause. After this and other moving happy reports, conflict arose again during the introduction of Zorida, a new client, because of her criticism about the state of the bathroom. Marcus jumped in to chastise the group, saying: "Although the house is closed, people still doing the same shit they were before—the stuff that got them here in the first place. Although they supposed to be clean, they still actin' dirty." Many clients nodded in agreement, appreciating his double entendre. Being off drugs did not make you "clean" at WTS: what mattered were other behaviors, including the willingness to condemn fellow clients and expose oneself to public shame, something Tiffany and Whitney did not do.

This meeting captures some of the complicated dynamics among clients. While I had little access to their more private interactions, I found that this mixture of support and conflict was common. WTS claimed to want women to support each other, yet its practices of surveillance intentionally undermined these connections. During a meeting of the "Gettin' Honest" group, Brenda discussed getting in trouble for touching another woman and making her uncomfortable. She defended herself by claiming that she had been trying to make friends. Walter, a counselor, condemned this, but not because Brenda had violated her peer's wishes. "Where did you get the idea you were here to make friends?" he retorted. "There are no friends in treatment." Because of the pervasive surveillance and the way clients were pitted against each other, living at WTS could be volatile and treacherous. Several clients complained to me that they didn't trust fellow clients. While this technique is useful for maintaining control, studies of correctional institutions show that encouraging distrust among women prisoners can be emotionally damaging.[38] Because everything about the self is part of addiction, penal rehabs like WTS wholeheartedly embrace informing. The complete lack of privacy accentuated the punitive aspects of treatment.

CONCLUSION

Advocates of treatment hope that by adopting the disease concept of addiction the criminal justice system will not only become more effective at controlling drug use, but it will also reduce the stigma of addiction and help address poverty. WTS is committed to working toward these goals, but to do so staff members must develop working definitions of addiction to determine women's needs. Like most of the treatment industry, the program's constructions of addiction have little to do with medical theories. Medical authorities emphasize the impact of drugs on the reward systems of the brain, but for WTS and the state agencies that mandate women to treatment, addiction is much bigger than uncontrolled drug use or behavioral deviance: it is women's disordered, weak selves. For WTS staff members, women's dependency explains all of their clients' problems, including drug use, poverty, failed relationships, and violent victimization. It is the women, not the penal state, who are addicted to punishment.

Viewing crime, family dysfunction, and poverty through the lens of addiction reveals a distinct framework of state governance. It is not only a shift from the warehousing of mass incarceration, it also differs from traditional versions of rehabilitation and welfare provision. Certainly, therapy has a long history in correctional institutions and in addiction treatment. And there is no doubt that penal and welfare agencies sought to change behavior, morality, relationships, and individual psychology. However, at WTS addiction reconfigures long-standing disciplinary techniques with new definitions of what is wrong with deviant women and different ideas about what women need to be independent, productive citizens. WTS's version of addiction draws from punitive discourses about criminals and the black poor and reformulates them through gendered and racialized definitions of addiction. As a result, WTS did not see work, sobriety, or following the law as measures of normalization. The work that mattered was on one's dependent self.

WTS staff members genuinely believed in the goal of making the legal system more humane and helping criminalized women overcome racial, class, and gender oppression. Other studies of women-centered penal treatment show that WTS is part of a larger trend of programs oriented toward the self and trauma.[39] However, WTS is unusual in the wide range of vocational and social services it offered, making it a best-case scenario of what reformers want from penal rehabs. In a remarkable move, WTS even bused some clients to the state capital to advocate for drug law reform with legislators. Yet these structural and political critiques had little influence on how staff members defined addiction or interpreted women's needs. Staff discussions of clients show that the trope of addiction consistently blinded the staff to the social causes and consequences of poverty and marginalization. Governing through addiction individualized inequality by subsuming marginalization inside the self. When the self is the problem, women are responsible for their own degradation. Staffers never recognized their role in the penal system or the echoes of racist and sexist stereotypes in their construction of addiction because WTS, like other gender-responsive programs, "position[ed] itself as a reprieve from structural forces."[40]

Scholars of TC-style penal treatment programs for women are especially critical of the way they ignore experiences of gendered abuse and rely on racist constructions of addicts. In contrast, WTS relies heavily on gender-responsive theories about sexual violence and women's enforced dependency. However, WTS replicates precisely the same racial, class, and gendered constructions of addiction that McCorkel found in a punitive, prison-based TC where women were regularly called crack whores.[41] In this chapter, I have argued that penal rehab programs are punitive and stigmatizing not because they do not attend to gender, but because they are punishments. WTS shares with Gladstone Lodge and many other institutions the use of disciplinary and normalizing techniques that seek to make people self-regulating. However, backed by the state's power to punish, these techniques were extremely coercive and stigmatizing at WTS. The program's construction of addiction depended on racialized discourses about crime and the dangerous, permanently dysfunctional poor. While it operated in the name of curing dependency, it fundamentally relied on the curtailment of autonomy. When Christine, who was profiled in the introduction, had an abortion to "focus on myself," she used program language to explain her decision. But she also made that decision because Marcus had told her she would be expelled if she did not. The prison and the system of mass criminalization underwrote treatment at WTS, even when women adopted the program's rhetoric. As a punishment, WTS's definition of addiction imparted the stigma of a criminal record, and in doing so, it reinforced racial and class boundaries.

CHAPTER 3

Women's Treatment Services

HABILITATING BROKEN WOMEN

IN ONE LONG, HOT CASE REVIEW meeting at Women's Treatment Services (WTS), Rachel, a counselor, reported on one of her clients, Belinda. Belinda was "not coming from her gut" during their counseling sessions because she was consumed with worries about her son. Rachel told the other staff members that Belinda's son was having behavioral problems in school, but the grandmother who took care of him did not speak English and so could not advocate for him to receive extra services from the school. According to Rachel, Belinda was "frequently emotional," blamed herself, and wanted to "step in." We learned that Belinda had asked for permission to visit the school and get him help. After Rachel said this, another staff member commented that Belinda should "focus on her self first before advocating for her child." Naomi, a younger black counselor, suggested that they determine whether Belinda's distress was due to "her guilt" or a "real problem of the son being underserved." Another staff member asked who Belinda was, and once Rachel described her, the staff's speculation about Belinda's state of mind turned to what she had been wearing. Several staff members jumped in to observe that she always wore a large, dumpy, beige sweater. They collectively deduced that this must be a sign of emotional problems—probably issues with her weight. This prompted a few staff members to note that they that had seen her eating at odd hours. One suggested that she had a problem with compulsive eating. In the end, the staff decided that Rachel would contact the school to see if the problem was "real." Belinda was forbidden from intervening. The staff also agreed to take Belinda off kitchen clean-up duty, to which they had previously assigned her as punishment, to keep her away from food, and Rachel resolved to ask Belinda about her body image in their individual sessions.

What most worried the counselors in Belinda's case was that she seemed focused on her son and not on her self. Because WTS viewed addiction as the result of a disordered and dependent self, Belinda's feelings about her child were seen as distracting her from the important feelings, those about her self. Staffers encountered this problem often. It was the most common refrain that I heard while observing them discuss clients. The majority of women at WTS were interested in reinvigorating relationships with their children and other family members.[1] Many had become estranged from their families while they were in prison or using drugs. Those who had cases with the city's child protective services (CPS) agency also had to demonstrate their fitness as parents. Some, like Belinda, just wanted to remain involved while in rehab. But at WTS, these desires—like women's interest in work accomplishments—were signs of codependency because they involved fulfillment outside the self. Therefore, WTS staff characterized women's desires to care for others as symptoms of addiction. In fact, Naomi showed skepticism about whether the problem with Belinda's son was "real" and suspected Belinda of projecting her problem onto her son to avoid dealing with her self. As the staff talked, they found what they believed to be Belinda's real issue, one inside her self: body image.

This chapter charts what habilitation—the remaking of women's selves—entailed at WTS and explains why women's social relationships, especially with their children, were seen as a barrier to their recovery. First and foremost, habilitation meant focusing on the self, which required clients to go deep into the therapeutic process of self-discovery and uncover gut-level emotions. Consequently, counselors needed intimate knowledge of clients' pasts, and as I will show, they required women to disclose painful emotions and chart their family pathologies. WTS's ultimate goal was to produce a new, more autonomous and self-reliant woman who becomes self-managing by needing very little from other people. For the counselors, Belinda's codependency, guilt, and low self-esteem were manifestations of a gendered form of addiction. To habilitate what Yvonne, director of WTS's Legal Services Department, once called "broken women," WTS sought to reform the gendered aspects of their lives and selves, including motherhood, sexuality, and embodied presentation of self. This meant that WTS clients had to distance themselves from their existing social ties. In addition, WTS also sought to make over clients' appearance. Thus in the name of transforming the self, WTS pushed women to change their clothing, consumption, and grooming.

These techniques reflect a larger trend toward understanding the harms of gender and racial oppression through psychological and self-help discourse about codependency, trauma, and addiction. Accordingly, Belinda's problem was not a lack of responsibility or a failure to live up to traditional gender norms. In fact, she was too beholden to the norm that women sacrifice themselves for their children. WTS counselors recognized that gender relations constrained women, for instance by making Belinda feel guilt as a mother and shame about her weight. But for the staff, the primary effect of this subordination was on the self, and its main toll was on self-esteem. There is no doubt that poverty, abuse, and social marginalization cause very deep wounds, including trauma and low self-esteem. However, WTS's logic systematically transformed clients' diverse and complex problems into therapeutic ones. As a result, the solution to Belinda's situation was more intensive counseling, a shift in the disciplinary structure in which she lived, and a change in how she dressed. At the next week's case review meeting, Rachel followed up on Belinda: she had admitted that she felt bad about gaining weight. Rachel also confirmed that Belinda had been removed from kitchen duty, but she never mentioned Belinda's concerns about her son. WTS's addiction framework did not enable the staff to think about gender as it intersected with class, race, or ethnicity. I argue that this therapeutic response to inequality renders invisible the social and material constraints on women. By forcing women to abandon family and social engagement, it also suspended their citizenship. As a result, it held women responsible for their own marginalization and often reproduced the very disempowerment that the counselors hoped to challenge.

WORKING ON THE SELF

When Lucy, a counselor, talked about her client, Tamika, she described her as "compliant." The staff obviously disapproved of rule breaking, but compliance could also be a problem. In this case, it showed that Tamika was dependent. She had been in treatment before and did well in the structured life of a rehab program, but once she was on her own she "lost it." To further illustrate her dependence, Lucy explained that Tamika is in a same-sex relationship but does not see herself as lesbian. This comment provoked a discussion. Apparently, Tamika had suggested that the relationship was about comfort. As the group of staff members talked about her, they came to see her rejection of the term "lesbian" as a sign that she was not comfortable with her own choices. Lucy decided that Tamika had "no relationship with her self," a sign of codependency, which would lead her to relapse when not in a structured environment. Lucy wanted to teach Tamika to develop her own structure, but her decisions about her sexuality did not count. She had to build a "relationship with her self." Habilitation aimed to create new selves by breaking women's dependencies, removing their old identities, and teaching them more autonomous forms of self-fulfillment and meaning. In worrying about whether women like Sofia, Kate, Charlene, and Belinda were avoiding their selves and resisting treatment, the counselors were fretting over whether women were engaged in the practical techniques used to "work on" and shape the self.[2] Through these techniques women learned about themselves and put their lives (and their problems) into WTS's narrative of addiction. The counselors hoped this labor for self-knowledge would produce greater autonomy.

"Getting Gut-Level"

In the first session of the parenting class, Karen, the family therapist, wrote "mother" on the blackboard and asked the clients to go up and write words they associated with it. Helping each other with spelling, the women wrote "love," "nurturing," "home," "bathe," "breastfeed," "togetherness," and "trust." One woman wrote "missing them," but basically all the words were positive— representing the idealized mother role. Then Karen went up and wrote "guilt" on the board and the staid, classroom-like atmosphere in the room suddenly disappeared. The women nodded in recognition, sighed, and said "oh!" Then the more difficult feelings came up: shame, abandonment, heartache, and sadness. At the end, the blackboard was completely filled. That day Karen led a tearful discussion about the words and the students' guilt and shame about being bad mothers. The discussion centered on wrenching confessions: Ella, a black client near forty, described smoking crack incessantly to try (unsuccessfully) to induce a miscarriage and her guilt for putting the baby at risk. Several women described having their children taken away at birth because of a positive drug test. Another confessed to stealing from her kids. Isabel, a thoughtful Latina woman in her twenties, described with great pain how her former boyfriend had called her "worthless" and refused to let her see her daughter. During this discussion, Karen sympathetically told the class that mothering is often hard and stressful, and filled with feelings of inadequacy. In the couple of weeks that followed, the parenting class continued to focus on confessions of guilt and shame. Only then did Karen move along to teaching practical parenting strategies.

Confessions about painful experiences and feelings were the centerpiece of focusing on the self and a primary activity of treatment. WTS expected women to divulge all of their most personal feelings to their counselors and during group sessions with other residents. Karen referred to this as "getting gut-level." These confessions were then subject to analysis by both clients and staff members. WTS used these confessions to reveal to women that their problems were the result of an addiction to punishment. Habilitation came through this self-knowledge, which staff members hoped would enable clients to construct a new identity, freed from their baggage and able to govern themselves. Clients' experiences of rape, sexual abuse, prostitution, family strife, and grief were crucial fodder for the staff meetings. The program's diagnostic process would not work without this knowledge. Consequently, they interpreted a woman's refusal to disclose events in her life or her emotions as an insuperable obstacle to recovery.

Making this kind of confession freely and genuinely became a marker of success; progress in treatment was often measured by whether women had disclosed painful emotions like self-loathing and revealed traumatizing experiences. Once Karen reported on a client whom she said was not "getting gut-level" in their individual sessions. The woman was close to her discharge date but had done badly on a test to move up a level in treatment. Karen noted that the only thing the woman talked about during counseling was her mother, but they had been over this ground before. Karen concluded that the woman was using these overly superficial confessions as a way to avoid some deep underlying issue, and Rachel agreed. However, Patricia, the director of the Restabilization Program, was skeptical. She asked what more they expected, since the woman had been in treatment before. What if she had dealt with her issues? Why should she always be crying and "delving into some drama"? Finally, Patricia briskly told Rachel and Karen that issues with your mother are "enough" to have a drug problem—"not everyone has been raped." This disagreement shows that it was not always easy to determine what kinds of emotional hurts sufficed and whether clients were confessing every dark part of their past. As a result, counselors often pushed women to raise the stakes of their confessions.

When I walked into Donisha's contentious case conference, she was sitting at the end of a long conference table opposite five staff members. The tension in the room was unmistakable. Donisha was upset at the critical progress report WTS had sent to her judge, which she said made her look like a "fuck-up." The staff was upset that she had written a letter to the judge asking for early release, which Yvonne told her looked bad. Donisha was angry because they did not want her to speak for herself. She defended speaking on her own behalf by saying that there were "things I didn't do even when I was druggin', and I'm not gonna start." To explain the critical review, Rachel gave the example that Donisha resisted treatment by not "disclosing" to her counselor (Lucy) when she refused to write her life history, including descriptions of her childhood, family life, sexual abuse, and drug history. Donisha defensively explained that she didn't remember details due to a brain injury. Yvonne attempted to calm the situation by asking Donisha to talk with her counselor to jog her memory. Donisha responded indignantly that her counselor wasn't working for her, but the staff refused to switch her to another counselor, saying the problem was with her, not Lucy. To illustrate this, the staff pointed out that she had failed in treatment three times before. Angered, Donisha explained why she had left other programs: at one place a male resident had assaulted her, and at another vindictive staff members had called the cops, who had violently shackled her.

To redirect the issue back to Donisha, Rachel gave another example: Donisha did not discuss her feelings about having her parental rights to two children terminated while she was in prison. The staff told her that disclosing these feelings would indicate her good progress for a pending family court case to regain custody of her remaining child. Donisha confidently responded, "I got that," to convey that she had dealt with this issue and did not need to go over it again. She went on, "I cried for seven years" about it, but now, she repeated, "I got that." Yet to prove she loved her kids, Donisha said that she would try for "five years" to get back custody of her infant daughter. With this, she argued that she knew how to deal with the loss: she had a plan and did not need to talk about it. The tension escalated as Donisha defensively gave explanations in response to each criticism. Some staff members said, "I hear you" a few times, but Jay, the WTS court liaison, chuckled and shook his head whenever she spoke. Eventually, Donisha refused to respond to him. In the end, the staff threatened Donisha with discharge if she would not follow the treatment plan. They also reminded her that the judge demanded that she open up to her counselor, and that this was the only way she could reunite with her daughter. Donisha retorted that she knew she'd lose any chance of regaining custody if she was "kicked out." Staff members tried to spin this coercive situation as an example of how she would benefit from doing what they asked, but Donisha still refused to write a life history and insisted that the staff respect her.

Donisha wanted to draw boundaries between herself and WTS by refusing to discuss certain things and by writing to the judge on her own behalf. Given her limited agency, she resisted WTS's power through asserting a different sense of self based on having privacy and advocating for her own interests. Donisha was not the only client who resented the staff's characterization of her as weak and dependent. She saw herself as a survivor. Meanwhile, the staff interpreted Donisha's resistance through the codependency framework, seeing it as a sign that she was avoiding dealing with her self, rather than as an indication of laudable independence. It is notable that while the staff members expected her to feel pain related to mothering, they saw getting gut-level as her only legitimate response. Moreover, they were able to use their legal power over Donisha's CPS case and her feelings for her daughter to press her to confess.

This kind of intense addiction treatment depends on the significant power the penal state grants WTS, including its long treatment times and, as was the case with Donisha, coercive power to break up families. A few years after completing my ethnographic research at WTS, I returned for a follow-up interview with Yvonne, who had been promoted to residential director. She explained that WTS had had to speed up the introspective process—at least for some clients. This was because parole funding had shifted to a "performance-based" system. Instead of getting funds in a block grant, WTS now gets small amounts of money for each milestone a client meets. These "contract goals" are set by the state parole agency and include the client's receiving an orientation packet; completing an intake interview, a screening tool, and a psychosocial evaluation; attending specific groups; passing out of the beginning orientation level; and then finding employment. If a client is a day off the schedule, WTS does not get the funds. "They not playing," Yvonne remarked.

"Everything happens very early now," she lamented. Yvonne regretted that "we can't sit for hours and go over it all" with the parolee clients. WTS's practices thus reflected the program's commitment to gender-sensitive treatment, a model that has only gained traction in penal rehab field since my research. Yet the state shaped the form treatment took and the speed with which clients had to get get-level.

Staff members expected clients to get gut-level in nearly all groups at WTS, including didactic sessions (such as the parenting class) and vocational groups. Clients should be ready to disclose at nearly any moment. This constant level of emotional exposure is painful and exhausting, so some women only pretended to get gut-level, and staff members policed clients' disclosures for authentic emotions. This made confession obligatory, continuous, and public.[3] As I slipped into the back of the "Gettin' Honest" group, the women in the crowded room were going over a sheet about family patterns and discussing how families pass on substance abuse. Linda, a counselor, asked Jenea, a young black client, to talk. With her jaw set and in a hostile tone, Jenea mumbled something vague about her mother's death. Linda loudly chastised her, "Jenea! Stop being gangsta and feel this!" Other women in the group laughed after Linda called Jenea out. Spurred by this mocking, Jenea began to eloquently explain why she had to be tough; she was the "mother to [her] mother." She grew more animated as she gave examples of having to carry her mother out of crack houses when she was ten years old. Verging on tears but still sounding hard and angry, Jenea spat out that her mother did not "do that for me." She began to cry in earnest when talking about how she had cared for her mother. "No one else in my family would *touch* my mom." Jenea then divulged how let down she felt that her mother had died and was not there for her as she'd promised. During this dramatic and moving confession most women in the group began listening intently and nodding. One client energetically responded, it's like "you told my life or something," and then went on to speak about her mother's death. Linda looked triumphant and vindicated at Jenea's tears, happy about this intense, honest, and unexpected outburst from a "gangsta" client.

Many therapeutic techniques ask participants to engage in introspection to understand the self, one's motivations, and how past experiences relate to behavior. At WTS getting gut-level was essential because it developed and transmitted WTS's narrative of women's life histories and current situation. For Jenea this meant not being "gangsta" any longer. This governing technique provoked powerful emotions as women disclosed painful feelings and embarrassing events. This stressful process worked to invest women in the program, sometimes by simply wearing them down and other times by using their empathy, as when Jenea became animated and encouraged others. It also served as a way to test clients' honest investment in treatment. Moreover, it helped staff members understand where to target their treatments, providing tools to plan their work. Linda ended the "Gettin' Honest" group by telling the women that it was possible to change these patterns by recognizing and understanding them. This was another important technique of self-transformation at WTS.

Identifying Patterns

Following confession, clients had to identify patterns in their feelings, family dynamics, sexual histories, drug use, and other behaviors. Through activities like the life history Donisha had to write, clients followed the mandate to "focus on themselves" and so developed a sense of themselves as consisting of these disordered patterns. When I arrived for one parenting class, Ella, usually expressive and upbeat, sat looking depressed and disheveled, without her typical styled hair and dressy clothes. She had recently absconded and relapsed after seeing her estranged daughter, who had been angry and resentful. During the discussion in class, Ella got gut-level. She wept and said that she wasn't ready to deal with her daughter yet. Karen nodded kindly and told Ella that she was right. She wasn't ready for mothering, Karen explained, because she had not worked through her "guilt and shame." And if she did not do so, these feelings would always be a "path" back to using. Ella pointed out that she had talked about these feelings in this class. Karen responded that she could tell that Ella had "not processed" this stuff because she had used drugs again. Moving into her gentle didactic mode, Karen asked the group "how do we process this stuff? We say 'work through the guilt' all the time, but what do we mean?" An awkward silence followed, and finally another woman suggested that they should forgive themselves and not live in the past. Karen noted that regret is part of being human and encouraged Ella to make lists of all the things she had done as a mother that caused her to feel guilt so she would learn her "triggers." Karen explained that the list would help her "process" feelings through recognition of the patterns connecting emotions and actions.

In parenting class, Karen typically addressed women's issues with their children by connecting the clients' experiences with their parents. Through the process of emotional confession WTS staff hoped that the clients would adopt the program's methods of understanding themselves. As we went around the circle during one class, one client mentioned that she felt guilty because she was not there for her kid, just as her addicted mother had not been there for her. Karen explained this through the statement "sometimes families have patterns that get passed down" and asked the women to talk about their own childhoods. Several students in the class adopted the method of understanding the self as shaped by family pathology. Roxanne volunteered that her mother had died of a heroin overdose. However, in the next class, which was also about guilt, Christine resisted WTS's dependency narrative when Karen pointed out similarities between her life and her mother's. Instead, Christine blamed her "bad choices," using the language of responsibility to challenge the addiction framework. To convince Christine of the existence of patterns, Karen gently adopted a geological metaphor for the self as composed of "layers of sediment" that include the surface level of conscious choice and deeper causes. Treatment, Karen said, is designed to get at the deep layers—that's "what we mean when we say gut-level." Christine looked skeptical but remained quiet, and Karen moved on.

By teaching clients to understand themselves in terms of pathological patterns and feelings, WTS aimed to align their sense of self with the program's narratives and to produce new subjectivities. This technique of knowing the self was important because it organized gut-level feelings and connected them to relationships and addictive behaviors. As is the case with most therapeutic work on the self, clients were supposed to govern themselves with this knowledge.[4] In Linda's "Relapse Prevention" group, the clients had to fill out worksheets designed to identify patterns, titled "Identifying Relapse Warning Signs," based on the premise that there is a "beginning, middle, and end" to relapses. The sheet said that identifying warning signs would enable them to "turn back" before relapsing—to govern their desire for drugs. While checking off their "triggers" from a list of possible warning signs, such as spending "less time with program friends," "being overly confident," and "avoiding problems," one client joked that WTS was her trigger and even Linda laughed. After everyone announced what she had checked off, each woman had to develop a plan to correct herself when she noticed a sign and share this plan with the others. At the end of the group, they all signed a "helping hand contract" to agree to monitor each other for these signs and intervene. Making an inventory of one's patterns was supposed to produce a new sense of self based on internal motivations rather than external sources and so develop an autonomous self-concept. As the "helping hand contract" suggests, therapeutic processes were intertwined with the group dynamic of the residential setting. Confession, self-management, and monitoring others were interlinked parts of the habilitation process and institutionalized in WTS's client hierarchies and surveillance.

CRIMINALS WHO LOVE TOO MUCH

WTS's gendered techniques of habilitation rested on codependency discourse. Originally, codependency described the psychological condition suffered by family members of alcoholics, whose lives were consumed with managing another's addiction—the family members are *co*dependent. It is now a much broader category. Codependency is a "primary disease" of excessive dependence on others, not just a by-product of having a relationship with an addict.[5] It operates as the source of all addictions—what the sociologist Leslie Irvine calls a "master addiction."[6] According to this framework, women's close relationships, self-awareness, and self-esteem were the major targets of treatment. Submerged in codependency's generally apolitical discourse is a therapeutic way of challenging women's traditional obligation to be dependent on men and responsible for care work. This critique of gender relations was important to WTS staff members. Through codependency, they invoked gender far more often than race or class, which were featured in WTS's official literature but rarely mentioned in everyday life. Therefore, WTS used ideas of addiction to interpret and ameliorate the gender constraints that their clients faced, while downplaying the racial and class constraints.

Joyce, an after-care counselor, had good news about Isabel. She was in the process of breaking up with her boyfriend, Bruce, with whom Joyce said she was "codependent." Isabel was a repeat client who had absconded from WTS once before. According to staff members, she had done so to be with a man. Isabel was allowed to return once she claimed she had become committed to herself. She had just successfully completed the residential part of the program. Karen, who had taught Isabel in the parenting class, exclaimed "that's great" after she heard the news. Joyce noted that "you can see the maturity level." Karen replied that "she's beginning to rely on herself." Agreeing, Joyce said that Isabel is beginning to "identify who she is." Greg, her vocational counselor, said that Isabel had always been "using or in relationships . . . [and] not taking time to get to know her self." In one way, they infantilized Isabel by commenting on her "maturity." But Greg's comment indicates that WTS had a critique of gender norms. Habilitation was not just about producing docile conformity; instead, it was part of a project of freeing women from gendered subordination. I do not know what Isabel's relationship with Bruce was really like or whether it was oppressive, but for the staff, her move away from him was not only a path away from drugs but also one toward equality.

As a feminist researcher, I was intrigued and impressed by WTS's gender politics. The program's narratives seemed to run counter to most of the derogatory mainstream characterizations of poor, nonwhite women who use drugs. However, over time, I saw that WTS's approach to gender is quite stigmatizing and punitive. According to WTS, it is ultimately women, and their supposedly innate tendency to be more "relational" than men, who are the problem. As the title of one best-selling codependency book puts it, they are *Women Who Love Too Much*.[7] Take, for example, how WTS approached violence against women. As Yvonne emphasized previously, trauma was a key part of WTS's definition of addiction. The program was responding to a very real pattern. WTS reports that 75 percent of its clients have experienced physical abuse, and 60 percent have survived rape or incest, much higher than the rates for women overall. Indeed, I was regularly shocked and saddened by the sexual violence I heard about in women's life stories. Despite WTS's sympathetic recognition of this suffering, the trauma narrative constructed women as weak and disordered, rather than as survivors. This had punitive consequences. For example, counselors often gave women "emotional ages," to suggest that they had not matured since they had been assaulted. This happened to Ebony, whose father had raped her repeatedly when she was a child. Her counselor reported that Ebony said she preferred relationships with women because she couldn't bear to be with men. Marcus, the residential director, then declared, "This woman is emotionally about twelve to thirteen years old." WTS's website describes its clients as "followers," trailing men into the criminal justice system. While acknowledging they were victims of abuse in childhood, the website concludes that by the time the women arrive at WTS, most of their wounds are "self-inflicted." Hence, the trauma framework was a key part of the program's construction of the women as addicted to punishment. In a penal institution, this idea conferred great stigma on women like Ebony and legitimated WTS's intensive control of its clients. Through WTS, the criminal justice system holds Ebony responsible for managing the consequences of her own rape. Since addiction was what produced the mandate for her to go to WTS, she was, in essence, being punished for having been victimized. The stigma of dependency affected all aspects of women's selves and social relationships—especially those that were gendered.

Motherhood and Family as Pathology

As Belinda's case suggests, WTS did not just problematize women's sexual and romantic relationships. While all residential rehabs seek to remove addicts from bad influences, WTS demanded a radical kind of separation. Because WTS staff members believed that their clients suffered from dependent selves, they were suspicious of clients' investment in relationships with their children and other family members. In the process, WTS challenged many of the social roles and identities that undergirded clients' preexisting sense of self. The whole idea of habilitation suggests that there is little of value in a person's existing life. Moreover, the codependency framework locates the ultimate cause of addiction in excessively needy relational ties. This stigmatized care work and all forms of interdependency because they are associated with women. Consequently, WTS urged women to distance themselves from their families so they would shed their codependency and create a new self. While clients had to talk a lot about their family relationships in therapy, they were not supposed to have much to do with their relatives. This was why

WTS pushed women into single-room-occupancy facilities (SROs)—staff did not want them to move in with their family. The addiction framework suggests that to challenge gender inequality, women must combat their weak ego boundaries and become more individuated.[8]

In case after case, WTS staff members presumed that women's family relationships were pathological. Malia got in trouble for bailing her brother out of jail while she was out on a pass to leave the facility. When Walter, her counselor, reported this incident, he said that Malia was proud of how she had handled this because her family could rely on her in a crisis. She thought she'd been on top of things. Malia had called her mom in the South and gotten her to wire money for bail. At each step she kept WTS notified about what she was doing and that she'd be late. Walter noted that it was particularly important to Malia to be dependable because she no longer had custody of her children. Despite this, Walter presented the incident as a bad sign for her. Malia shouldn't be taking care of others' problems, he said. It is notable that Walter did not fixate on the fact the Malia had broken the rules of her pass. His concerns focused on what Malia's "deviation" meant for her self. In this way, he conceptualized her problems as separable from her role in her family and her family's problems. Moreover, Walter's account downplayed the context that made Malia's actions meaningful: losing custody of her children and all the associated stigma. Thus, WTS reduced all of women's issues to their addictions.

Staff members believed that caring for others was not only a trait associated with women's addiction, but that caring for others while in treatment prevented women from caring for their selves. As a result, mothering in particular posed a threat to women's recovery. In one meeting, Rosa, a Latina counselor, reported on Marlena, who had just transferred from WTS's Residential Program to its outpatient day treatment program. Rosa informed us that Marlena was pregnant and had not told anyone at WTS until after the transfer. The room let out a collective gasp and erupted in chatter. Women at WTS are not allowed to be pregnant. Not only did the staff frown on women's having sexual relationships while in treatment, but if a woman decided to continue her pregnancy, she usually had to leave the program. So if Marlena wanted to stay in residential treatment at WTS, she would have to get an abortion.[9] While Christine was confident that ending her pregnancy was the right decision, as discussed in the introduction, Marlena did not want an abortion. Rosa reported that Marlena claimed to be "happy to be a mother again" and was determined to regain custody of her other two children, who were in foster care. To Rosa and her colleagues, however, Marlena's desire to have a baby and her shrewd request for a transfer signaled a lack of commitment to treatment and to her self. They were offended by her hubris, and she no longer seemed eligible for a transfer to the outpatient program. Rosa declared that

Marlena was "focusing on children rather than her self" and looked to men "for validation." Exasperated, Rosa concluded that Marlena was just "using" WTS for services, including help getting her general equivalency diploma (GED) and a job, without "learning anything." The others concurred with Rosa that Marlena was avoiding treatment and decided that she needed a case conference. Once Marlena showed a lack of willingness to work on her self, Rosa put Marlena and her irresponsible childbearing into the trope of the welfare queen.

WTS did not typically admit pregnant women. This was partly because it did not have the space or licensing to house and care for children. However, during my fieldwork there, one pregnant woman was allowed to stay because her due date was after her discharge date. Nevertheless, Maria caused a lot of anxiety and conflict. When I first heard Marcus, her primary counselor, report on her, he rolled his eyes and sighed dramatically. He was having "nightmares" about her having the baby at WTS, he said. He noted that he was trying to get her discharged as quickly as possible. But Maria did not want to leave. He explained to us that she had never lived on her own before and was nervous about it. Marcus warned his staff that he knew she had been trying to convince some of them that she had permission to have the baby there. Marcus stated that they could not admit pregnant women ever again. Marcus accused the staff of coddling her because of "countertransference." He claimed that they were working out their own "issues" about not caring for their children by going easy on Maria, prompting Patricia to mutter that she was not. Marcus also made a big deal about how they needed to make sure that Maria moved far away from WTS. He noted with glee that Linda, the after-care counselor, could visit her all the way on the other side of town. Marcus then told the staff to make sure Maria did not return with the baby and declared with finality that women couldn't have babies at WTS. One staff member laughed at the idea and exclaimed, "They'd all be having babies up in here!" To reiterate his point, Marcus stressed, "We are a treatment facility!"

A month later, I heard Linda report on how Maria was doing after she had left WTS. Maria and her new son—named after Marcus—were living in a terrible apartment that was indeed on the other side of the city. It had no heat and no hot water, so it must have been quite cold because it was only early March. The owner was a slumlord, Linda said. She resolved to help Maria find a new place and search for jobs. Linda also mentioned that Maria wanted to return to visit WTS. The staff, however, wanted to keep her away from the other women. Marcus called WTS Maria's "umbilical cord" and advocated that she not be allowed to visit. This language vividly constructed her as dependent and immature. Linda was working to improve Maria's living situation. But the staff did not consider the relationship between Maria's wish to stay at WTS and the lack of social and financial resources that landed her alone, in an apartment with no heat or hot water, while caring for a newborn and recovering from a cesarean section. Maria's pregnancy rendered WTS's treatment methods untenable. This went beyond the facility's legal inability to house children: Maria's obligation to care for her baby did not fit with WTS's ideal of the actualized self. By constructing her as overly dependent on the program, the staff transformed their bureaucratic need to discharge Maria into her psychological need to become more autonomous. It was common for staff members to turn organizational needs into clients' needs. In the end, the attempt to cure Maria's dependency left her in dire straits, with little support to care for herself or her son. Despite its veneration of autonomy, WTS faced challenges actually getting women to achieve this special state.

During a break in the meeting, I asked several counselors why Maria had caused such problems for them. Rachel told me that when Maria had been living there, she had heard other clients say things like, "I can't wait until I get pregnant again." Rachel mimicked her response, "But you in treatment! Why you talking about having a baby? How can you be thinking of having a baby?" She explained the clients' reaction as a desire to make up for being absent in their kids' lives. The next week, Patricia told me something similar. I mentioned that I had noticed that issues related to children were common among the clients. She set out to explain why, saying that many women had not been in their children's lives: "They get sober for twenty minutes, then they decide they want to be parents." Referring to clients' ongoing struggles with CPS and the family courts, Patricia argued that the courts look after the kids' interests. They are not against the mothers per se, she noted, but the women don't always realize this. Like Rachel, Patricia attributed clients' parental desires to their feelings of guilt for failing as mothers. In addition, she pointed to cultural pressures that make it obligatory for women to mother, even if deep down "they don't want to." It's okay not to want to be a parent, even if you're a woman, she explained. Patricia clearly worked to counter this gender norm in everyday life. She was frequently dismissive of effusive fondness for children and often made positive comments about women who were childless.

Addiction and the Politics of Motherhood

Staff members were quite aware that women are expected to meet the impossible standards of "intensive mothering" and were stigmatized if they did not sacrifice themselves in this way.[10] Although this was never spoken out loud, they were also aware that clients' race and class augmented their stigma, especially that related to motherhood. WTS staff turned to addiction discourse to challenge this racialized and gendered shame and to help women manage it. Rachel once asked her colleagues for advice on how to deal with Rhonda, who felt tremendous guilt about what she had done in front of her children. With audible sympathy, Rachel noted how intensely Rhonda beat up on herself. Everyone on the staff then agreed that Rhonda should not feel bad because she had been powerless in the face of her addiction—her actions were not intentional. Patricia argued that Rhonda "doesn't understand the disease of addiction," so she needs to go back to the first of the twelve steps and admit her powerlessness.[11] They also concluded that Rhonda was too focused on her guilt and was spending too much time trying to make herself look good to her kids. She could not move beyond this to work on her self in treatment. To stop Rhonda from focusing on them, Rachel made plans to bring her children in for family therapy. The addiction narrative may have eased her guilt and family counseling is probably useful, but the staff members asserted that the root of the problem was Rhonda's dependence on outside sources of self-worth.

Yet WTS was not uniformly hostile to motherhood. Like the rest of American society, staff members were navigating unresolved tensions over gender relations, family structure, and women's roles. Therefore, they were ambivalent about motherhood. So when Maria did end up visiting, she received a very warm welcome, just as Marcus had feared. When she came in the front door Ayana, an intake specialist, and Joyce rushed up to hug her, squealing and excited. They jokingly cooed, what happened to your belly? Maria was beaming. They asked her where baby Marcus was and how he was doing. As Maria stood by the doorway, still more staff members dashed up to say hi and hear about the baby. When Yvonne finally returned to her office, she tried to shift back to seriousness by explaining that Maria could not bring the baby to WTS because he had not had his vaccinations. Yet Yvonne could not conceal the thrill of this exuberant, warm moment.

Staff members were less critical of their own families and parenthood but remained ambivalent about them. WTS held a boisterous and festive, staff-only baby shower for an administrator, Pamela, who was going on maternity leave to have twins. The dining room was decorated in blue and pink streamers, and everyone was there, joking, eating cake, and playing silly baby-themed games. Someone asked Rachel whether she was going to have any more kids, and she emphatically said no. She was "closing up shop" and said "the factory shut down." Three is enough in this day and age, Rachel concluded. When the guest of honor arrived, Yvonne referred to her as "all three of you." Pamela said that she had been dilated 1.5 centimeters two weeks before, and the room erupted in chaos. Yvonne, hysterical with laughter, put two small bowls at her feet. Ayana grabbed napkins; someone else broke out plastic gloves. Marcus referred to Maria and joked that Pamela had to get out. "No babies at [WTS]!" he teased. During the toasts, Marcus described how his now-grown twins never go away and are still hitting him up for money. Janet, a counselor, told Pamela that good and bad times lay ahead but also emphasized that children are a blessing and so Pamela was doubly blessed.

Clients also expressed a range of emotions as they struggled to balance the demands and promises of autonomy with the value of connection. At house meetings, clients had a regular segment devoted to good feelings. Children, family, and friendship were common themes. During one meeting, a client named Danielle stood up and, with her voice full of emotion, said that she had received a picture of her son. She had never seen him as a grown-up before. Although Danielle wasn't happy that he was in prison, she was ecstatic to hear from him. He wanted to see her for the holidays. The other clients were genuinely happy for her, clapped vigorously, and asked to see the photo. Another woman got up and announced that she was going to go to school and would get her GED in January. We clapped. The next client, Camille, said that she had been clean for seventy-nine days and was doing better at WTS. "I was stressed about my kids, but now I am less focused on that, and I know who I am, and can spend time on myself. Today is a good day," Camille said. She got enthusiastic applause. Zorida stood and said she had been clean for only a week, but at least she was sober and had her "sisters' help," referring to the other clients. Next, another woman rose and stated that she was glad for another client who had helped her face her addiction and realize that she still struggled with it. She said she was glad to be sober and was taking it one day, one minute at a time.

Feminist scholarship suggests that WTS's ambivalence about dependency, care, and gender has deep historical roots in a political system that values independence as the basis of citizenship but also associates these traits with men and with paid labor.[12] Codependency discourse reworks this veneration of autonomy to include women and to emphasize emotional instead of financial or political self-sufficiency. Yet it also condemns women for not living up to their potential independence. WTS is not unusual in adopting this framework. Nearly every study of a North American correctional institution for women in the past fifteen years has reported they assume that women are overly dependent and need to focus on themselves.[13] When researching women's self-help books, the sociologist Arlie Hochschild found the codependency framework juxtaposed against a more conservative narrative of what women need, according to which women benefit from patriarchal family relations and find happiness by caring for others. While not a fan of the traditionalists' love of male dominance, Hochschild is also critical of the codependency framework for "abducting" feminist concerns about women's oppression in the home, while maintaining the antifeminist devaluation of care, interdependence, and emotion.[14] Likewise, WTS's conception of addiction had the effect of devaluing things associated with femininity and thus stigmatizing clients as women. This echoes popular and political tropes that demonize drug-using women of color for both being unfeminine and lacking personal responsibility. WTS did not offer a way out of this tension between femininity and autonomy. For example, CPS removes children from women's custody if they do not meet expectations for responsible mothering.[15] This placed the WTS clients with CPS cases in the awkward position of having to demonstrate their ability to be a responsible mother while also meeting WTS's demand that they not focus on their children. They were caught between two competing standards for women, which were impossible to fulfill together.

It is certainly the case that there are cultural pressures on women to meet unreasonable mothering standards. But rather than focusing on how women could negotiate these relationships while also finding time for themselves or helping women learn to resist unfair expectations from family members or lovers, WTS simply asked women to disconnect themselves from these relations. By demanding separation from family ties and constructing women as pathologically dependent, WTS's approach reflects long-standing state practices and racist beliefs that devalue black motherhood, children, and families.[16] While they tried to combat women's shame and guilt, WTS staff members often characterized the clients as reckless breeders because they were so dependent. With its emphasis on the self, the addiction framework blinded staff members to the way that women's experiences of racism, poverty, and punishment shaped their attachment to mothering and family life. Yet Patricia Hill Collins has shown that in a world that devalues black lives, mothering can be a form of resistance for African American women.[17] Moreover, research on women who are incarcerated or poor shows that they often use motherhood as a way to find dignity and meaning amid limited opportunities—even as mothering and related gender ideals also constrain them.[18] However unlike black feminist scholars such as Collins, WTS staff members found it hard to acknowledge the value of women's families while also recognizing how gendered family arrangements can be oppressive. Instead, the staff asked women to relinquish the need for recognition from others and to rely on themselves to feel good.

PENAL MAKEOVERS

Near the end of a three-hour staff meeting, Patricia speculated that one client was having a "gender identity crisis" due to her changes in clothing from "butch" to "femme" and back again. This juicy topic gave the group of ten or so staff members a second wind and prompted a long, engaged discussion. A few initially asserted that this client was gay. Two others noted that they had never seen her dress femme, while one counselor claimed she was just being unisex. Many concluded with Patricia that the client must be confused.

Linda, who was out as a lesbian and dressed in somewhat masculine clothing, argued that the client was simply dressing based on what she could get from "the Boutique," WTS's stash of donated clothes. Another staff member suggested that these changes in dress meant that the client was bisexual, which led Patricia to triumphantly reiterate that the client was confused. Annoyed, Linda argued that bisexuality was legitimate and didn't mean that she was confused. At this point Greg and Margaret, the social worker, interjected that the staff members were working out their own issues, and that the conversation was not about the clients. Only then did the speculation cease.

Another aspect of reforming women's gender focused on their appearance, grooming, mannerisms, and presentation of self—in short, how they "do gender."[19] Counselors frequently drew on women's appearance to figure out what their issues were, as they did with Belinda. In this example, Patricia felt that the client's changing fashion signaled a deeper confusion in her self. Her gender presentation should be coherent and should signal her sexual orientation. While the staff members disagreed about how to interpret the meaning of the client's clothing, such discussions were common at WTS because staffers tried to uncover the deep psychological issues that they believed caused women's problems. In addition, the program sought to foster new practices that encouraged women to "take care of the self" through feeling beautiful. These penal makeovers targeted gendered aspects of what Pierre Bourdieu would call habitus—embodied, class-linked dispositions and ways of acting.[20]

Yvonne explained, "You take the broken women, just like a little plant. . . . You start nurturing them, give them good information, tell them when they look nice." She told me that when clients first arrived, staff members removed the women's degrading prison-issued orange sneakers: "That's the first thing that has to go . . . because it's too much of a reminder of where they've come from." Yvonne marveled at the rapid transformation clients made. As the treatment changed their inner selves, the results showed in women's hair, nails, and clothing. Yvonne would compliment them: "Wow, you got makeup on. That's nice!" She explained that other treatment programs force women to dress very blandly, but she was proud that WTS encouraged women "to take care of the self." It "is the one thing that helps them to build their self-esteem." Normative femininity was therefore an expression of the real self's breaking through years of abuse.

At WTS, habilitation required learning to "take care of the self" in decidedly feminine ways. On my very first day at WTS, the deputy director proudly told me that WTS had a "spa day" when women received makeovers, facials, and manicures. It was, she said, "the best day." During one meeting of Janet's regular group called "Encounters with Self," an esthetician from a fancy salon came in to provide the women with facial skin analyses. She took a good look at their skin, told them what type it was (such as "dry"), and recommended beauty products. At the end, the esthetician raffled off some facial products. Many women in the group seemed to appreciate her helpful tips on moisturizing, but the session was about more than fun. Reforming women's appearance and consumption taught women to rely on themselves, not on other people or drugs, to feel good. This technique sought to create a capable, autonomous feminine subject through gendered self-care. Much as the clients were asked to discuss their family dynamics and govern themselves with this knowledge, Janet hoped the esthetician's exercise would teach abused and stigmatized women to know, value, and manage themselves. Cultivating the self, outside as well as inside, was an important step toward recovery. Framing gendered consumption as a form of healing from sexism and racism suggests the truly commercial aspects of "commercialized feminism."[21] Nevertheless, it also makes learning normative (and potentially costly) ways of consuming beauty products part of a criminal sentence.

Consumption was integrated into WTS's system of rewards and punishments, serving as a disciplinary technique as well as a way to shape subjectivity. When women first arrive, they cannot leave the facility, so the program supplies them with toiletries. If a client does well, she earns the privilege of going outside to shop, first at a corner store and then farther afield, a technique that fosters women's independence through consumption. Yet this freedom required a lot of management. Counselors often discussed how to stop their clients from spending too much on grooming products or their children. At times, clients used consumption to resist treatment, such as when several women got into trouble for getting manicures without permission. Disciplinary consumption also generated conflict. Women in the more restrictive, nine-to-twelve-month Residential Program resented that the clients in the three-to-six-month Restabilization Program could access their money and go shopping almost immediately. Donisha, who was in the Residential Program, explained to me that it was especially insulting that Restabilization Program clients could buy their own food. Conflicts over shopping, consumption, and grooming were common during house meetings. Being able to control one's consumption was important to clients, who used it to defend their sense of self from stigma. During one smoking break, Luisana said she loved going to the store because it made her feel "normal." She liked "being myself" and on her own. "I want out!" Luisana yelled to nobody in particular. While we were talking, a young black woman came out, looking like she had been crying. She complained to us that because of some infraction she had been forbidden to go to the store that day to buy cigarettes. She then counted all the smoking breaks she would have to go through with no cigarettes. Another client took pity on her and gave her a cigarette. More than an addiction, smoking was a moment outside the program, both literally and figuratively.

Women's participation in this physical transformation indicated their willingness to leave behind their old lives—especially their old identities— behind. One day, I ran into Roxanne, a white client around forty, while walking into the building. I asked how she was, and she emphatically said "lousy!" She hated WTS—it was driving her crazy. Roxanne exclaimed that Walter, her counselor, was "such an asshole." He took some of her money from the savings WTS kept for her and told her to buy a dress. Roxanne often wore tight T-shirts, jeans, and sneakers, and Walter told her that she was "an older woman" and should not dress that way. This infuriated Roxanne. Venting, she told me she did go to the store, but all the dresses there had flowers or stripes on them. Roxanne said she didn't like flowers or stripes, so she hadn't bought a dress. "Isn't it my prerogative if I wear a dress or not?" she asked. "They can't tell me how to dress! . . . The thing that gets me is, it's my money!" I asked if the dress was for work, thinking that must explain Walter's instruction. But no, Walter had told Roxanne she was not dressing the way a woman her age should. When she returned without a dress, he called her "grimy."

Walter sought to make sure Roxanne was not invested in the identity of being a sexy young woman. Although Yvonne encouraged women to look and feel beautiful, being too sexy was bad because it showed a woman's dependence on other people for her sense of self. I followed Roxanne into the building where, in tears, she retold the story to Ella. Roxanne recounted that other clients teased her by saying Walter was in the right because she "plays with him"—that is, flirts. She lamented that she couldn't take WTS or "these bitches. I feel like I'm going crazy." Ella was outraged on Roxanne's behalf and called Walter "unprofessional." Moreover, she made the case that Roxanne dressed "young" but not "sleazy," and that her outfit was within the WTS dress code. Concerned that Roxanne would abscond, which as a parolee could land her in prison, Ella asked her to talk to another counselor and reminded the HIV-positive Roxanne that she needed to take care of her health: "You can't do that in prison; you don't get anything there."

Ella's comment about the "pains of imprisonment" shows the coercive backdrop against which this gender and class disciplining took place.[22] To Ella, getting health care was what it meant to take care of the self. But when clients became resistant, Yvonne would ask "Do you still have those orange sneakers?" to remind them that WTS gave them access to a femininity that the criminal justice system took away. Staff members genuinely hoped beauty services would make women feel worthy, yet by attempting to recuperate women's femininity WTS depended on the very stigmas it was trying to undo. Reforming women's appearance managed them in ways that seemed gentle and gender-appropriate. It was a vital part of what made WTS women-centered.

Yet this strategy disguised the coercion involved in penal treatment and rein-scribed the idea that gender deviance caused the women's problems.

WTS was trying to make a particular type of woman, one who would be able to resist the pitfalls of poor, racialized womanhood. Staff discussions focused on the class and racial meaning of women's gender presentation. I frequently heard counselors report that they were "working on the client's loudness issues." During a meeting, Marcus updated the staff on a difficult client. She had recently been restrained for getting angry while meeting with her parole officer. When Marcus said she was "childlike" and "loud as ever," several women on the staff affirmed in unison, "uh-huh!" He was "working on" the client's "self-presentation" and "voice control." Although being loud was bad, so was being passive. Patricia once called a client "histrionic" because she "played the victim," blamed everyone but herself, and walked with her head down. Seeming to be lower class was problematic—for example, Linda criticized a client for speaking "street" at a job interview. Sexually provocative clothing was also an issue, and one woman was criticized for wearing stiletto heels to her remedial classes. In addition, the staff often mocked women's con-sumption of food. For one "peer day," the clients decided to go to a local park for a picnic. Donisha was tremendously excited about this and told me that women were saving up to buy batteries for the stereo and food. She did not know that in the meeting where the staff members voted to approve this out-ing, they had laughed uproariously about the amount food the women would eat and how many coolers they would have to take. Some even imitated how the clients would walk while overburdened with so much food.

WTS wanted women not only to be self-actualized, but also to be proper ladies. During the annual graduation ceremony, one graduate spoke to the audience of clients, their family members, and staff members about her recov-ery. She praised WTS counselors because in addition to enabling her to "for-give myself," they had taught her "to dress like a lady." By taking her to plays and museums, WTS had given her "social skills" that she had not had when she was "out on the street" and "animalistic." Staff members' concern over things like loudness, "ghettoness," and "streetness" were part of the same mis-sion. Through these gendered transformations staff members sought to rid women of gender presentations that signaled racial marginality. Thus, these makeovers were also a way of trying to manage clients' race and class status. There is no doubt that staff members wanted to make their clients more acceptable to employers, judges, and other authority figures. Vocational and legal assistance was a formal part of the treatment process at WTS. However, Walter's instruction that Roxanne buy a dress reveals that employment was not the primary goal. When Margaret reported to her colleagues about a client who desperately wanted to get custody of her children in foster care, she was dismayed that the woman had showed up late and improperly dressed at family court. Making a bad impression on the judge was a reasonable concern. However, Margaret shifted her understanding of the woman's mistake from one of following the norms of the court to a therapeutic framework. Margaret put the client's inappropriate clothing in context by noting that the woman vacillated from being childlike and tearful to being withdrawn and aggressive, and that she touched Margaret's leg every time she disclosed something. Margaret resolved to "work on her clothing," her "dislike of consequences," and her lack of "boundaries" and "independence."

It certainly is beneficial to have cultural skills that help in negotiating bureaucratic institutions, and since WTS had little ability to affect the labor market, changing the women was about the program's only option. But by framing the problem as psychological, WTS constructed fitting into the middle-class, white world as a sign of having the proper relationship to one's self. Cultural capital can help people succeed, especially in formal settings like courts and job interviews, and therefore such unstated rules of behavior reproduce privilege. The education scholar Lisa Delpit argues that people from marginalized communities benefit from being taught these rules explicitly.[23] She notes that well-meaning, privileged whites often misread direct, top-down instruction in culture as illiberal authoritarianism. However, at WTS, women's problematic self-presentation was not seen as deriving from their social disadvantages. Nor did WTS pitch changes in appearance and language as strategies for successfully playing the mainstream game. Staff members approached women's self-presentation as a sign of psychological issues. They did not acknowledge that these norms are the (ultimately arbitrary) cultural codes of those in power, as Delpit suggests. Consequently, habilitation rests on the construction of racism, poverty, and legal troubles as individual psychological problems.

Historically it was common for correctional programs to try to reform women's femininity.[24] Class- and race-linked ways of "doing gender" were thought to be causes of women's deviance and poverty. In an odd echo of the progressive era, I heard many staff members report that they were "working on" a client's "hygiene" or, in more contemporary parlance, "independent living skills." Staff members' efforts to reform women's presentation of self are also part of a long tradition of black racial-uplift movements.[25] Often led by middle-class African American women, these movements have sought to improve the condition and social status of blacks through encouraging various forms of respectability—including gendered ones. The movements' tactics included not only education but also changing dress, speech, sexual practices, and household management. Like the racial-uplift advocates of the progressive era who helped develop the juvenile justice system for African American youth,[26] WTS's leaders wanted to integrate personal reform into the penal system. Setting a good example was important. On the day of the baby shower Yvonne was wearing tight jeans, high-heeled boots, new hair extensions, and a revealing top. Standing in front of the room of revelers, Marcus teased her by calling her "Foxy Brown," thus racializing her provocative outfit. With humor, he said he had to explain to the clients that she was dressed for "after-work, not work." Yvonne and Carl teased him right back, pointing out that Marcus regularly wore mesh shirts and a gold chain with a cobra's head on it to work.

Unlike most twentieth-century racial-uplift movements,[27] WTS did not see the patriarchal family as an ideal model. Giving women makeovers, like creating distance between clients and their families, aimed to "empower" the women to find fulfillment in themselves. At one graduation, WTS clients staged an exuberant fashion show wearing professional-looking clothing. This was partly a hopeful message about upward mobility. However, the executive director's message to the graduates drew heavily on codependency discourse when she described upward mobility as a psychological process. She stated that "self-love" is way to resist "racism, classism, and sexism." The graduates "have chosen responsibility over sabotage and self-destruction" and "chosen to . . . walk in [their] own power," thus "overcom[ing] their addiction to pain and punishment." In this document, the executive director suggested that improving addicted women's self-esteem is a radical act that challenges oppression. Yet at the same time, her message suggested that clients' social disadvantages were largely of their own making. This apparent paradox is the result of conceptualizing the damage inflicted by racism, classism, and sexism as primarily within the self and using the penal system to ameliorate that damage. At WTS, changing women's gendered selves became the solution to problems of inequality, governing gender as a way to manage class and racial marginalization.

CONCLUSION

WTS is part of a long history of institutions that seek to control women's deviance from gender norms.[28] While its addiction ideology bears the mark of contemporary culture, WTS still constructs women's gendered deviance as the cause of their legal deviance. Again and again, researchers find that attempts (whether penal or medical) to control and reform women focus on sexuality, the body, and mothering. WTS is no different. Habilitation targeted the gendered aspects of women's selves and lives. Because definitions of deviance are often gender-specific, practices of social control operate differently for women than they do for men. Simply being a criminal is more deviant for women, because crime is considered masculine. The same is true for drug use and drinking. From popular culture to political discourse, women who take drugs—especially women of color—suffer additional stigma because they are depicted not just as addicts or criminals but also as failed women.[29] Most WTS staff members recognized this. In addition, the problems they worried about, from guilt and unreasonable family demands to trauma, were very real and concerning issues for many clients. Yet the addiction framework prevented the staff from effectively challenging the notion that women who use drugs or break the law are deviant as women.

Nonetheless, addiction discourse does change how penal institutions construct and govern poor, nonwhite, and criminalized women. WTS's ideal woman is not the docile service worker one would imagine a workfare program might promote, or the modest and attentive housewife venerated by correctional institutions in the past. She is an autonomous therapeutic subject, who is empowered by needing nothing but herself. There are costs to this ideal. Studies have shown that the transformation of a stigmatized, addict identity is a central aspect of the recovery process. People must adopt a nonaddict identity, and they need social and institutional supports to acquire and maintain these new identities—what sociologists call identity resources.[30] They must rely on either old or new socially valued identities to shed the addict stigma—for example, getting involved in work, family, or political causes. In other words, people need a narrative of self and the social resources to underpin it. WTS was not especially good at providing women with these resources. While I do not have traditional outcome data to track relapse or recidivism rates, the process of habilitation actively sought to undermine women's existing identities while replacing them with an identity that by definition had no social supports at all. Especially with limited access to careers, pervasive racism, and the stigma of a criminal record, the women at WTS were left with little but introspection, consumption, and makeovers to build a new self.

WTS staff members and advocates of gender-sensitive treatment hope rehab will counter marginalization through empowerment. However, feminist critics of empowerment programs argue that they depoliticize gender. WTS does not quite support this argument. Instead, it did politics therapeutically. Barbara Cruikshank argues that within such therapeutic logics "the political is reconstituted at the level of the self."[31] Empowerment politics rests on the idea that social relations should provide everyone with self-esteem. Staff members hoped that reforming clients' gender would counteract the effects of oppression on self-esteem, but WTS paradoxically pathologized women further. What WTS's empowerment efforts failed to do is recognize the social and economic basis of women's subordination and its intersection with racial inequality. This is because the program's addiction recovery discourse relied on a false dichotomy between dependence and autonomy. Feminist scholars have long noted that classic ideals of autonomy are premised on women's dependence on men and the exploitation of nonwhite groups.[32] WTS deployed this model of autonomy, and within it women must go without social support and avoid care work. This model of treatment aligns with the penal state's larger patterns of social abandonment.

WTS's punitive and stigmatizing dynamics reflect the fact that it is a punishment. For years, many scholars argued in support of therapeutic responses to incarcerated and drug-using women.[33] Treatment, they hoped, would address women's true, socially based needs. Instead, I found that WTS reframes the effects of gender and racial inequality as matters of addiction and then holds women accountable for managing them, using the threat of harsher punishment. This produced the strange situation in which the state uses punishment to make women love themselves. Gender-sensitive addiction discourse thus extended the power to punish. However, WTS's practices of confession, makeovers, and separation from family reflected presumptions about the value of clients' prior lives and selves that cannot be made so easily in the case of more privileged women. What happens if you take treatment out of the penal system? In the following two chapters, I turn to Gladstone Lodge to examine what happens when women-centered rehab is not a punishment.

CHAPTER 4

Gladstone Lodge

MARISOL ARRIVED AT GLADSTONE LODGE because of what the staff calls "job jeopardy." A working-class Puerto Rican woman in her fifties, Marisol is a member of a utility workers' union and lives in the same city where WTS is located. When she arrived at work smelling like alcohol, her supervisor pushed her into treatment. So Marisol headed to the Lodge. Like many of its clients, she had been in treatment there before—twenty years earlier, in her case. During one daily group devoted to learning about the twelve steps of Alcoholics Anonymous (AA), Marisol's turn came. The day's topic was the tenth step, which requires making a regular inventory of one's progress and flaws.[1] Marisol first described how she would spend her workday planning her drinking. Then, at length, she emotionally recounted that her mother was cruel and controlling. After a while, Betty, a counselor's aide, interrupted to move the discussion along. Later that day in the case review meeting, Marisol's counselor, Joan, asked "Is she sharing?" Betty exclaimed, "Yes! I didn't think she'd ever stop sharing." Moreover, Marisol wasn't even talking about the tenth step or her drinking. Joan noted: "She definitely has issues with her mother. . . . I don't know if I could live with her [mother]." But later, Joan raised a concern, "She's got a real entitlement thing." Betty added, "She don't shut up, I know that."

Two weeks later, as Marisol's time at the Lodge was drawing to a close, it was her turn to "tell her story" to the other clients. All women at the Lodge have to do this once. In contrast to most groups there, women's stories get very personal. Marisol began with her extremely abusive parents. She was denied food, beaten, and left unwashed. Her father made her kneel on raw rice for hours, which caused excruciating pain. Marisol earned admission to a school for the gifted, but her mother would not let her go because Marisol did all the cleaning, cooking, and child care at home. Marisol's mother also prevented her from having friends or boyfriends, took the money she earned, and forced her to have a harrowing illegal abortion. It was a heartbreaking story, but after Marisol spent a while tearfully recounting the abuse and describing how she felt unloved, Joan leaned in to instruct her, "Talk about your drinking." Obligingly, Marisol explained that she started drinking while waiting for her (now former) husband to come home from his affairs. The drinking got really bad after Marisol found out that he was sexually abusing their twelve-year-old foster daughter. She finished her story by saying that she had a pension and wanted to get sober so she could enjoy retirement.

Marisol's story contained just the kind of gut-level anguish, trauma, and codependency that was at the center of Women's Treatment Services' (WTS) approach to addiction treatment. However, counselors at the Lodge consistently felt that Marisol was too fixated on these issues. Instead, Joan pushed her talk about her drinking. While WTS used its enormous power to force women to get to the gut level, Betty wished Marisol would "share" less. It is not that the Lodge counselors were unsympathetic. Moreover, they believed in gender-responsive treatment and encouraged the clients to draw on these discourses to understand Marisol's experiences of abuse. After hearing her story, two clients immediately noted that she was "codependent" with her mother. For example, Donna said: "We addicts, we don't have boundaries. We weren't taught boundaries." "It's time to take care of [Marisol]," other clients urged. Joan agreed. When discussing Marisol with her colleagues, Joan was horrified that she had been "used as a slave" by her mother and suggested that Marisol change the locks on her door to keep her mother out. In the end, however, Marisol's drinking mattered most.

Joan redirected Marisol's story to her drinking because the Lodge defines addiction as chemical dependency—not a weak, diseased self.[2] Staff members knew that women faced other difficulties, but their job was to treat addiction, and for them this meant getting people clean and sober. The Lodge consistently framed substance abuse as women's most pressing problem. Joan explained to Marisol that "your mother's always going to be there, going like this" and made a talking gesture with her hand. This, Marisol could not change. What she could do was stop drinking. For the Lodge, sobriety required social and moral rehabilitation, not habilitation of the self. In the discussion after Marisol's story, the solution offered for her loneliness and drinking was not to focus on herself, it was "you gotta go to AA." The staff arranged for Marisol's union representative to drive her home that week. He was reportedly a "hard ass" about going to Narcotics Anonymous (NA) or AA. Mary, a senior counselor, hoped the fact that he was a "handsome Hispanic man" would help to charm Marisol into relying on the twelve-step community for help.

This chapter examines why Gladstone Lodge constructed addiction as substance abuse, how it understood the goals of rehab, and why its approach was so different from the one used at WTS. Annette, the Lodge's clinical director and sole social worker, explained that "for us, it is about chemical dependency." This different notion of dependency meant that treatment acted on the self but did not require a wholesale transformation of it. Recovery required learning to live sober. While WTS women were expected to change their selves, Lodge women were expected to change their lifestyles. There are two interrelated dynamics that underpinned the way Gladstone Lodge constructed addiction and carried out treatment. First, being in the health-care system constrained what the program could do. Although many clients were in job jeopardy, the Lodge lacked the coercive power of the penal state. Health insurance pays for only short stays and does not fund any of the services that enabled WTS to bring all of women's lives into addiction treatment. Mary argued that these time limits made it impossible to deal with individuals' deepest issues. She explained that it takes "time to put people back together again."

In addition, Lodge staffers did not think that their clients needed to transform their selves. The Lodge purposefully avoids state funding and the criminal justice system to get people who the staff thinks are the best addicts, ones who are respectable "working people" like them—including many police officers. Nearly everyone who worked at the Lodge was in recovery, and they were on a moral mission to save their fellow addicts. Bill and Faye, the husband and wife who founded and own the Lodge, wanted to defend their clients and their own precarious social status by offering "a haven for the chemically dependent." Marisol was not especially privileged by class or ethnicity, she had a very troubled family, and staff members certainly considered her to have an addiction. However, she was not tarred with the stigma of a criminal record or its racial and class connotations. Consequently, the staff saw her as a particular kind of addict, one in need of much less controlling and punitive treatment than that found in the criminal justice system. In contrast, treatment at the Lodge promised redemption from stigma and reintegration into society. After Marisol had recounted her story, she was told that she deserved a happy retirement.

THE PRIVATE TREATMENT SYSTEM AND THE NARROWING OF ADDICTION

Gladstone Lodge is based almost entirely on the twelve-step method invented by AA, which is typical of most private-pay rehabs. In the vast majority of group sessions, clients are asked to read aloud from a twelve-step text and apply its ideas to their own lives. Recovery in AA is a social process based on moral accountability and egalitarian fellowship, outside of medical authority. AA and its offshoots like NA spawned most of today's recovery methods—even those models that depart from twelve-step orthodoxy, such as codependency and therapeutic communities (TCs). But Gladstone Lodge is truly orthodox, what Don, its executive director, called a "vintage Cadillac." As Bill grumpily remarked one day, "I guess I'm old school." This means that some of the Lodge's terminology and practices would be recognizable to people with little knowledge of rehab. For instance, clients introduce themselves by saying, "Hi, I'm [name], and I'm an addict." They also must admit they are "powerless" over their "disease" and "surrender" to the process by putting their faith in a "higher power" and "working the program" "one day at a time." Readers who have spent any time in what followers of the twelve steps call "the rooms" (AA or NA meetings) would be able to sit down in a Lodge group and participate fluently.

The Lodge's twelve-step approach is far from medicalized. Rather, addiction is seen as a spiritual disease that functions somewhat like original sin. Individuals are born with this incurable condition, but it can be managed through a process that resembles religious conversion, one that scholars argue conforms to middle-class ideals of self-control and rationality.[3] It is this deprofessionalized, quasi-religious set of ideas and practices that underlies the Lodge's treatment. Scholars of penal rehabs like WTS assume that they are more exclusionary and subordinating than traditional twelve-step programs because they hold that addicts are different from normal people, that addicts are morally flawed, that addiction is a permanent condition, and therefore that addicts must surrender to regulation.[4] I agree that penal programs are punitive and stigmatizing. However, each of these beliefs is standard fare in AA and NA, and each is gospel at Gladstone Lodge.[5] Despite sharing some beliefs and practices with penal rehabs, the Lodge turned out to be a different—and less punitive—form of treatment. For example, Joan's correction of Marisol would never have happened at WTS.

Substance Abuse Is the Problem

For the Lodge, substance abuse is the cause of most clients' problems and a poor way of handling the rest. Annette told me that "we want them to start writing and looking at what the chemical dependency's done to their life, right away." Defining addiction narrowly as "chemical dependency" directed treatment away from the self and "getting gut-level" and toward getting sober. Addressing trauma is central to the theories of gender-responsive treatment, yet everyone at the Lodge disagreed. "The pain is the result of using," Bill explained. Following the AA adages of "easy does it" and "keep it simple," he warned against "too much deep stuff." When I interviewed Annette, she said, "We're not doing intensive psychotherapy, but we're giving them the tools to know what those feelings are, to keep [the feelings] from getting people to pick up [drugs] again." In other words, the Lodge's job was teaching people to stay sober, even if they had other issues besides substance use "People present us with just every horrible problem that a human can have," Annette noted. But "we only have them for . . . two weeks to a month. . . .You have to be able to open [a trauma] up, and then do the work, and help people close it up, and we don't have the time to do that, and we don't have the training to do it. That's very specialized work. And we're teachers, we're educators, we're counselors." Annette argued that this kind of therapy "needs to be handled by a real professional who can take somebody through the process and help them get out the other side." Her voice full of emotion, she said that otherwise "you could do terrible damage," because when people leave rehab, "their guts are still hanging out."

Mary agreed. Sitting in her shared office, we discussed Gladstone Lodge's approach and women's gender-specific needs. Mary is a white woman in her late forties and is as composed and serene as Ruth, the director of the women's program, is energetic and sassy. Mary is a stabilizing force at the Lodge. She told me that the staff focused on substance abuse and not on all the many other problems that women may have, especially not deep, painful issues. Mary suggested that substance abuse was the staff's professional specialty. They are trained to treat addiction, unlike psychologists or psychiatrists—who she noted are "not trained in it." To illustrate this division of labor, Mary pointed out to me that psychiatrists are terrible at recognizing addiction and often exacerbate it by prescribing drugs. If Mary thinks a client has unresolved issues, she will recommend that she see a therapist after she leaves the Lodge. Not only did work on the self require time, but Mary thought that these issues could overwhelm the real purpose of treatment. To explain the dangers, she told me that in the past the Lodge had brought in a woman to give presentations on domestic violence. The speaker was a survivor herself and would tell her story to clients, then lecture about the patterns of domestic violence and its underlying family dynamics. Mary said that the presentation was amazing and always brought up difficult feelings in the women. But after the speaker left, "we had to deal with the aftermath." Because of this distraction from substance abuse, the Lodge stopped bringing her in to speak. Sobriety came first.

Both Annette and Mary argued that insurance companies provide such limited coverage that the program's focus has to be narrow. Since one month constitutes a generous stay in rehab at the Lodge (as opposed to WTS's three to twelve months), they contend that it is both unfeasible and unethical to dissect someone's self. However, there were a few clients who stayed for three or four months, and a couple of "extended" clients remained at the program for years. The Lodge did not require these clients to get gut-level. Thus, length of stay was not the only factor in defining addiction as substance abuse. The program was also constrained by its position in familial and work-based social control. Habilitation at WTS was aligned with the penal state's tactics of punishment and managing marginal populations, but the Lodge was beholden to families, unions, and employers. These entities want rehab to fit women back into their existing roles. So it is against their interests to remake women's selves and dissociate women from their relationships.

Yet Mary's and Annette's comments reveal that their definition of addiction is more than an adaptation to institutional constraints. They thought getting people off drugs was the essence of addiction treatment. The staff didn't want to do it differently. I mentioned to Annette that the other program I studied spent a lot of time on the self, and she said you can do that in a TC. I asked if this kind of work was necessary for recovery. "No," she said "I would actually look at it the other way." Annette argued that people need to learn to live without alcohol or drugs before they are ready to for deep work on the self. In fact, some may "just be fine" without such work, as long as they are sober. Annette made sure to note that "we make it safe" for people to share their experiences and offer them support. But ultimately these problems mattered only to the extent that they were relapse triggers. Annette observed that "the other danger of that is allowing them to get too caught up in it and too focused on it and then they lose the whole program." For the Lodge, "the whole program" was about chemical dependency. Staff used this definition to interpret what women needed. Treatment was organized around an abiding sense that clients cannot make anything else better until they stop using. As a result, case review meetings at the Lodge typically took a fraction of the time they did at WTS. In fact, the staff often skipped the meetings. This practice initially frustrated me, because I had anticipated that the staff meetings there would be as revealing as they were at WTS. But I realized that the meetings' lesser importance demonstrated the Lodge's narrow definition of addiction. Counselors did not feel it necessary to uncover a woman's broken self or manage everything in her life.

The Lodge's approach to addiction can be seen in the one notable case where staff members believed a client did not have chemical dependency. Elsa was a Latina police sergeant. On a night when she had had one drink, she and her partner got into a dispute and the partner called 911. When the police showed up, they determined that Elsa was "fit for duty," meaning that she was not drunk. What is more, Elsa drank only occasionally and never used drugs. However, because of the mere presence of substance use, the cautious police department where she worked forced her into rehab. Given Elsa's minimal history of drinking, the Lodge staff did not consider her an alcoholic. While she had to attend groups, she was exempted from the ritual introduction and simply said, "I'm Elsa and I have a sincere desire to stop drinking."[6] Elsa was also given unusual latitude in other ways. Every morning a staff member does a "room check" of the clients' bedrooms to make sure they are neat and without contraband. The clients who occupy the room must be there, as must the client assigned the rotating role of "Mayor." When Elsa was Mayor, as a joke, she would kick in clients' doors yelling "room check" in an authoritative police tone, as if it was a raid. The staff found this hilarious, but no other police clients did such a thing. In contrast, when WTS got clients who were not heavy users, such as Charlene, the staff still considered them to suffer from dependent selves and did not treat them differently from other clients.

Although insurance time limits aggravated them, Lodge staff members were content with the program's focus on substance use. At one case review meeting, Ruth reported bad news about Pat, a white police officer and Lodge alumna: she had relapsed and was in treatment again. Ruth is an outgoing, working-class Jewish woman in her late fifties, with many years of experience in the treatment field. She also has a long relationship with the Lodge—a former drug addict, she had been in treatment there herself. Ruth seemed unfazed by Pat's relapse: "She probably drank a couple of days and went back into treatment. . . . She won't drink the same way again." Dana, a counselor, laughed and said, "She thought of you!" In fact, the staff proudly joked that they were ruining clients' future highs. Ruth warned the women that that they would always hear her voice in their heads when they relapse. Rayanne, a junior counselor and former Lodge client, often told the women that the Lodge really cared for them and would send them birthday cards for the rest of their lives. But, she noted, the cards would make them feel terrible if they relapsed. Many Lodge counselors had relapsed themselves, and staff members anticipated that most women would do so, too. Thus, they saw their job as changing women's relationship to using and teaching them what Mary called new "coping skills."

Mandated by Life

The Lodge's construction of addiction as chemical dependency follows the first step, which states "we admitted we were powerless over alcohol [or drugs, in NA]—that our lives had become unmanageable."[7] To show people, in Bill's words, the "hold the chemical has on them," staff members spent a lot of time convincing women that substance use was the cause of their problems. Once I entered the cloistered women's unit and found the cozy and homey living room, where most groups were held, was filled with chairs facing a chalkboard. Ruth was going to give a lecture. She began by asking the eight women present who "has tried to get clean before?" Everyone raised her hand, except a new, young client who seemed to be ill from withdrawal. "What happened?" Ruth asked. One woman volunteered that she had "switched addictions" to another drug. A second said, "I didn't work a program." Ruth responded: "People come here because of the consequences. . . . If there were no consequences there would be no [Gladstone Lodge]. . . . And that's okay—whatever you need to stay clean." She explained that to "keep using despite negative results" was a definition of "insanity." Ruth then engaged the women in an exercise to convince them of their "insanity."

Ruth asked the women to "go back to a time where there were no consequences. . . . How many years of consequences do you have?" Several clients asked questions about how to define consequences. Ruth explained they
should count from the first negative consequences that resulted from using. "If
you had years clean [and] decided to pick up (and it *is* a decision)," start from
the very beginning, with even small things like a hangover. She then requested
a volunteer. There was an awkwardly long pause before a confident-sounding
client finally said, "Thirty years. I was seventeen." After Ruth prompted her,
the woman explained what her first consequences had been. To which Ruth
triumphantly responded, "That might stop somebody normal!" Writing "30"
on the chalkboard, she asked for someone to add up the years, and I volunteered. As each woman gave her count and explanation, I added the numbers.
They eventually came to 159 years of "insanity" for the whole group. Ruth
wrote this number on the board and asked me to divide it. I announced it
came to just under 20 years per person. She drily pointed out that this was a
big number, as several women looked alarmed.

Lodge counselors often claimed that people come to rehab because of the
negative "consequences" of drinking and drugging, such as being investigated
by the local child protective services (CPS) agency or the threat of losing their
husband, job, or parental support. The counselors called this being "mandated by
life." The phrase plays on the typical distinction in the treatment field between
voluntary admissions and those mandated by the criminal justice system to illustrate to the Lodge's voluntary clients that they have to be there. While WTS
produced a fiction of voluntary participation through its language of "contracts,"
the Lodge produced a fiction of mandates to impress on clients how serious
their situation was.[8] Gladstone staff members tried to use these mandates to
secure both clients' compliance and their genuine investment in recovery. Rayanne once told clients that they "were mandated by life to come here . . .'cause
something must have been going wrong in yous' lives to end up at [Gladstone
Lodge]." Rayanne described the epiphany she had had one day sitting "right
here in these chairs." If I kept using drugs, she said, "I would die. I just knew."
Clients like Cody, a white crack user, concurred when she claimed that "death,
insanity, institutionalization, and recovery" were her only options.

The "mandated by life" fiction also combated stigma. It enabled Lodge
staff members to avoid distinctions among clients with different pathways to
treatment, especially those with connections to the penal state, such as CPS
cases or criminal charges. In one meeting Ruth brought up Alexa, the twenty-
year-old heroin user who was one of the few truly mandated clients. She
had been in rehab eight times, including two TCs funded by the criminal
justice system—which she described to me as the worst experiences of her
life. Lodge staff members were suspicious of Alexa because she had been in

TCs. She had a pass to leave the facility for a medical procedure, and although Alexa's mother was taking her, Ruth worried that she would get high. Alexa has done this at other rehabs, Ruth noted, and "her mother is a big enabler." She reminded her colleagues that Alexa had convinced her mother to bring her to a friend's house after she had left a detoxification facility. At the friend's house, she took heroin and arrived at Gladstone Lodge high. Ruth sternly announced that if Alexa took drugs, "I will have to report it to probation" and decided to schedule "nursing to give her a supervised urine [test]" after she returned—something that was not done regularly at the Lodge. Then her demeanor lightened and she laughed, "They think they're so slick." Ruth commented that Alexa had had the hubris to explain to her how she could get away with it. She would not get high while outside: "I'd just bring them [drugs] in." To which Ruth had retorted, "try that and you will be gone." One staffer thought that Alexa was doing well, but Mary was more cautious because Alexa had been kicked out of a TC. Exasperated, Ruth described how difficult Alexa's mother was: she screamed at Alexa when dropping her off at the Lodge and gave the staff attitude. This incident required Ruth to intervene and exclaim, "What's wrong with you!" In fact, Ruth regularly complained that Alexa's mother was the worst mother of a client she had ever dealt with.

Despite the concerns about Alexa's commitment, history of rule breaking, and codependent mother, the staff members' decisions reveal that they saw these issues within the framework of relapse. The priority was making sure Alexa did not use. Mary said that Alexa "needs to tell [the doctor] that she's an addict" so she wouldn't be given painkillers (which would count as using). Ruth declared confidently that she once had the same procedure that Alexa was to have, and she did not need pain medication. Staff members also strat-egized about how to instruct Alexa's mother to take her directly to the doctor and then back to the Lodge. Mary ended by saying that she thought Alexa might have been high on her first day there, but now that staff members knew her, they would be able to tell if she was high. They did not discuss Alexa's need to focus on her self or to distance herself from her mother. Ruth did not deploy the legal mandate from probation to press for access to Alexa's self. Pro-bation served as a sanction to control using. Alexa may have been mandated to treatment, but chemical dependency was her main issue. When Alexa moved from the TC to Gladstone Lodge, she became a different kind of addict—one requiring different governing techniques.

"The Cream of the Crop": Gladstone Lodge as a Class and Racial Project

Faye and Bill started the Lodge as a way of following AA's religious-like directive to carry the message of the twelve steps to others. They are on a

mission to offer a "haven" to fellow sufferers, so the personal and professional
are deeply entwined for them and for the Lodge's staff. Faye is a confident
woman of sixty-eight, and Bill is a moody and earnest man who seems all of
his eighty years. They refer to each other as partners and claim that they owe
their lives to AA. Bill was in the military and worked in trucking and insurance before going full time into the rehab business. Like a story from the TV
show *Mad Men*, Faye worked in advertising in the 1960s, moving her way up
from secretary to copywriter. She vividly describes not wanting a life like her
mother's and struggling to be recognized for her mind. It was the advertising world that started her drinking, and getting sober ultimately led her out
of that world. Faye and Bill had, respectively, around forty and fifty years of
sobriety when I first met them. Because of their impressive sobriety and the
haven they offered, Bill and Faye were venerated by their employees—many
of whom had been in treatment at the Lodge and all of whom had some affiliation with twelve-step culture. Staff members spoke about Bill and Faye with
such reverence that when they stopped by to meet with clients, it felt like a
visiting dignitary had arrived. This meant that Bill and Faye took on parental
roles in addition to being the bosses, which gave Gladstone Lodge a distinctly
familial culture. There was a reason why they lived on the property: the Lodge
was what Faye called "our baby." She told me that they had never managed to
have children but were leaving the Lodge as their legacy instead.

Much of the Lodge's organizational structure and its treatment methods
stem from this mission. Its reliance on private funding and employment-based
referrals was not simply a financial decision. It was a symbolic choice that
reflected the twelve-step approach and the way that Bill and Faye connected
this model of recovery to class and racial politics. As a result, the Lodge is
ideologically opposed to taking public funding, which includes everything
from criminal justice contracts to state grants and Medicaid. This stance was
a source of pride. Annette told me that not having state funding was "a very
good thing actually. Because we can . . . run the program the way we want
without a lot of interference in terms of regulatory demands." Every staffer
that I spoke to explained the official reasoning for this decision in the same
way. According to them, state funding requires that programs not mention a
higher power, and it prevents counselors from disclosing their own experiences with addiction.[9] Both of these practices are part of the twelve-step
tradition. Annette argued that while formal addiction treatment was not the
same as AA, the Lodge remains "faithful to the idea of using the twelve steps as
a guideline" because it is "a method of treatment that has historically worked
the best for most." The Lodge hires only counselors who are part of this culture.[10] Don, a middle-age white man who managed the facility's finances, told
me that you get a "gut feeling" about who will fit in, and "having insight"

from personal experience was more important than academic training. He explained that the Lodge "has been able to create something special, with one alcoholic talking to another." Indeed, staff members regularly talked about their own experiences with addiction and recovery. The rule was that it was okay to do so if it was "for the benefit of the patient." This technique fostered clients' and staff members' identification with each other, while giving staff members legitimacy and aiding their control. Laughing, Annette said it made the clients "less likely to think they could" put anything over on the staff: "You can't shit a shitter." The Lodge's links to the police, employee assistance programs (EAPs), and labor unions also mean that the program is embedded in networks of lower-middle- and working-class whites, and these links make it dependent on employers that believe in "save the man, save the investment." The staff is quite aware that this employment-based system forms a separate tier of rehab programs from those that serve the poor and criminalized.

"Park Avenue to a Park Bench"

The material and symbolic structures that support Gladstone Lodge and its mission are disintegrating. Changes in the treatment field, the health-care system, drug policy, and the social status of its clients have given the Lodge a pervasive sense of being embattled and in crisis. The facility's main entryway contained a bench that clients had painted with phrases. One always caught my eye: it said "Park Avenue to a Park Bench." While this overstates the socio-economic origins of most clients, its reference to downward mobility captures the class anxieties that underlay staff members' fear that the program might not survive as "a haven for the chemically dependent," the kind of place that can redeem working people afflicted by addiction. The treatment industry is becoming increasingly competitive, and the private-pay segment boasts more and more luxury programs, which offer things like spas and seasonal cuisine. These not only conflict with the Lodge's twelve-step minimalism, but Lodge staff members generally lacked the cultural capital to pull these amenities off. While the program's website advertises a low-carb diet and a commitment to holistic wellness, the only thing the Lodge actually did to accommodate these tastes was to offer a yoga class (taught by a follower of the twelve steps). At the same time, the Lodge faces deeper structural problems. Union membership has declined dramatically, and working-class people's access to stable work with generous benefits is increasingly precarious. As fewer employers see their workers as an "investment" worth "saving," EAP referrals to rehab have fallen across the country.[11] Bill once warned that "we're dead in the water" without the union accounts.

Over time, the Lodge has had to rely more on insurance and the rehab market than on its contracts with EAPs to get clients. This made the program's financial situation precarious, much like the situation of their clients. Bill listed insurance as one of the factors "ruining the [rehab] industry." As managed care limited the number of days covered, it contradicted the staff's theories of addiction. Staff members told me it takes about thirty days for any drug to leave the body, so people are barely detoxified when they are forced out of the Lodge. And only when they are sober did staff believe people can really change. Being part of the health-care system caused the Lodge massive financial problems after the nationwide recession in 2008. It led to reduced client volume and, most destructively, long delays (often of more than six months) in insurance reimbursement. Moreover, Bill and Faye lost a large amount of their investments, which they had previously used as a cushion in tight times. Because of this, the Lodge could not meet its payroll during part of my fieldwork there. Staff members were paid for only three days of their five-day week. Throughout my study period, the program barely had enough clients to fund it, a situation made worse by the state's ban on smoking in rehab facilities. The staff's sense of crisis only accentuated when a client in the men's unit committed suicide. In addition to causing a wave of sadness and self-doubt among the staff, this tragedy meant that the Lodge lost a major insurer and faced intensive scrutiny by the state's Department of Substance Abuse Services (DSAS) and private accreditation bodies.

What is more, staff members had deep misgivings about medicalization and felt that it threatened the "tried-and-true" twelve-step approach. Although the facility was part of the health-care system, Bill regularly lamented that "this used to be a grassroots movement." One issue was that the Lodge felt state pressure to professionalize. Don told me that "if [DSAS] had their way [we'd be] 50 percent social workers." But most concerning was the rise of pharmaceutical drugs to treat addiction (such as Suboxone). The use of these drugs goes against the twelve-step model, which prohibits all mind-altering substances. The Lodge will not use such drugs. It even resists administering other psychiatric drugs, because staff members believe that they cannot be accurately prescribed until someone is sober. Annette expressed this view succinctly: clients have been addicts for years, and their lives are a mess, so "of course you're depressed!" Clients are "situationally depressed," she claimed, but not necessarily clinically depressed. Staff members in the Lodge's women's unit were especially critical of pharmaceuticals because they think women are vulnerable to the abuse of medical authority. When Ruth reported on a potential new client whose drug of choice was pain medication, the staff was wary about taking her. To fill me in, Ruth said that there are "no pills on the men's side." But the women's unit gets many clients with "severe pain issues" who become addicted to painkillers. For a long time, she argued, doctors' response to women was "give them pills!" But women who were dependent on pain medications caused the Lodge problems. Joan exclaimed "Ding, ding, ding!" to indicate that it set off warning bells. Ruth explained that they had to get people sober, but "we are required by law to manage people's pain. . . . [Yet] we're not a medical facility."

Vincent, the head of admissions, claimed that insurance companies and DSAS wanted the Lodge to use pharmaceuticals because they are "evidenced-based" treatment. Doing so would benefit the program financially by making it easier to extend people's coverage, because monitoring medication is a legitimate medical reason for inpatient treatment. Despite this incentive, the Lodge resisted. Since many people take psychiatric drugs, this caused regular conflicts with the Lodge's clients and doctors. One woman was furious that the Lodge would not allow her to continue taking her medications and called her psychiatrist, who in turn screamed at her counselor that this was malpractice and grounds to sue. The women's unit staff members discussed this incident at a meeting, and because of the psychiatrist's pressure they agreed to administer the medications. Still, Faye was annoyed at the staff for this compromise of the program's purity. Yet sometimes the antimedication approach helped with the Lodge's appeal. Becca, a young white drug user from California, flew all the way across the country to go to the Lodge because she and her family did not want her "doped up."

Faced with economic and symbolic threats, Bill and Faye doubled down on the mission. When Ruth and I arrived at one weekly managers' meeting, the senior staff of both the women's and men's units sat crowded together in the conference room with Bill and Faye at the head of the table—not a common occurrence. They were berating the staff for problems with how the facility was run. Later, Ruth noted to me smugly that their complaints were about the men's program. Indeed, Faye held up the women's program as exemplary. First, their concerns centered on a recent theft and the fact that clients were continuing to sneak cigarettes. As they discussed procedures for room checks and staff communication, Bill regularly interrupted everyone with aggressive questions about why they weren't doing their jobs and then scoffed at their defensive, sputtering explanations. Eventually Bill and Faye accused the staff of having "lost the mission," especially the part about "caring" for clients and using the twelve steps. If they were going to work at the Lodge it had to be more than a job; they had to follow the mission.

Bill became increasingly angry and sad at the same time, pointing out how their approach had "lost ground to the behaviorists." Maybe they're right, he said petulantly, we should give up. He repeated several times that "it is easy to start something from scratch, but it is hard to keep what we got going." Faye was more practical and centered. She forcefully explained how the staff had to follow the Lodge's systems, which included making sure that a client was assigned the role of "Greeter" to introduce newly admitted clients. Having a genuine "fellowship" among clients was essential to the twelve-step approach. It could, Faye noted, help prevent deaths, ominously reminding us that addiction was a deadly disease. Bill explained that it was vital for the clients to do the fourth and fifth steps before they left, which requires taking a "moral inventory" of oneself and an admission of one's wrongs.[12] He also argued for the importance of small things, like telling people to keep their feet off the furniture. Faye asked, what does this say about your commitment to "our baby"? She wondered aloud whether their efforts to build a legacy were worth it if this was how the Lodge was going to be run.

I sat through many meetings like this during my research. In response to the precarious position of the organization and the people in it, the Lodge mounted a full-on defense of its treatment approach, which was more than a professional philosophy. It embodied a fading social order in which people keep their feet off the furniture. The staff members, especially those at the top, were passionate about their version of addiction because they tied it to maintaining their respectable social status. Faye worried about larger moral decline, commenting that "we're dealing every day with a new breed of people coming in who are full of entitlement, and know better than authority." Fatigued by this decline, Bill considered "bypass[ing] the health-care thing" and turning the program into a "spiritual retreat." Faye wondered if they should convert Gladstone Lodge into a nonprofit foundation "so it doesn't get tainted by the younger generation" after they die. What the Lodge did not do in response to its financial problems was link up with the penal welfare state. In fact, staff members saw the growing involvement of the criminal justice system in the treatment field as another threat.

Getting the Best Addicts

The administration of Gladstone Lodge was both a classed and raced project.[13] The program and the people in it occupy an increasingly insecure place in racial hierarchies as well as economic ones. Its institutional strategies of avoiding public funding and contracting with unions were attempts to seek out people who the staff felt were the "best clients," an idea that was filled with racial and class meaning. During our interview, Don claimed that other treatment programs were jealous of the Lodge because it monopolized the "best accounts," the unions. They were the best, he argued, because members had good coverage and jobs. Similarly, Bill argued that union members were the "cream of the crop" because of their good insurance, supplementary benefit funds, social stability, and pressure from employers to go to rehab. This distinction was not just about ability to pay, however; it was also racialized. At the Lodge, race and class served as proxies to identify which clients would be successful and thus to indicate their social and moral value.

Despite the Lodge's objection to state funding, the program did take Medicaid many years before my research. The Lodge withdrew from Medicaid after what Bill perceived as an unwarranted fine for improperly completed billing forms. Being under that kind of state supervision "wasn't worth the hassle," he said, even if they could "count on the money." By giving up Medicaid's payments, the Lodge lost revenue. But it was worthwhile because it kept the program pure. Bill invoked racialized stereotypes of an underclass culture of poverty when he complained about the "off the street" attitude, "gold chains," and clothing of the Medicaid clients. These people, he claimed, were "not highly motivated," acted as if they had a "right to entitlement," and were "just using the system." Receiving Medicaid—that is, being poor—became a sign of criminality, blackness, and welfare dependency. Bill and Don claimed that the employment-based contracts were more valuable than Medicaid because the clients entered under the coercive pressure of losing their job, which gave the staff leverage. However, coercive pressure could not be the only thing that mattered. The Lodge refused contracts with the criminal justice system, which provide as strong a coercion as possible. Yet I found that it did take some mandated clients, like Alexa. Refusing Medicaid turned out to be a useful way to make this distinction, even though it hurt the bottom line. It was, quite intentionally, a class- and race-based distinction.

Lodge clients were seen as respectable people, just like the staff. In contrast to those on Medicaid, Bill explained, "we were dealing with working people, not [people] on the public dole." They were from "a different mold." The notion that Lodge clients were "working people" came up over and over again. Bill and Faye tried to keep the price down and were proud that their program was affordable to "working people," but they did not want the unruly poor. In our interview, Faye told me, "We really wanna just help those that really want to live a civil life." This idea of "our kind of addict" was a racialized distinction even though the unions sent quite a few people of color to the Lodge. Their status as "working people" spared them from the interlinking racial and class stereotypes associated with criminalized drug users. The idea of "working people" is also a gendered trope. While I constantly heard the administrative staff use the phrase, the women's unit staff never did. Many of their clients were "only" the wives or daughters of the much-vaunted union member. The women's unit staff did not use the coded racial discourse of Faye and Bill or share their conservative politics; however, the counselors remained committed to their clients' fundamental respectability and the limited definition of addiction this implied.

Lodge staff members invoke precisely the same stereotypes that underlie the penal rehab system and WTS's construction of addiction. WTS and the Lodge work in the same field and, as a result, their staffs operate with many of the same premises and distinctions. However, the drug war and the criminal justice system's movement into treatment threatened the Lodge by putting it in increasing contact with people who have criminal records and, like Alexa, had been in penal rehabs. This prompted the staff to do intensive boundary work. "I shouldn't say this," Don admitted, but "the main distinction is between programs that take Medicaid and those that don't." Leaving Medicaid was one way to avoid marginalized people, but it was crucial to avoid the stigma of criminality. The staff was perpetually concerned that "jailhouse" culture was infecting the program. For instance, Ruth railed against the clients' refusal to inform her about rule breaking by linking it to the prison's antisnitching norms. Faye complained to me about a reform to state drug laws that would release people from prison into treatment: "Now we're gonna be careful . . . screening people getting out of jails. Because you're gonna have a different mentality person. You're gonna be taking drug dealers, who are just looking to come into a cushy treatment center. . . . I feel sorry for government[-funded] programs because they have to be geared up for those people." Never a fan of what she called "big government," Faye complained that the reform would "build up another reason to put government programs in place for the people who suck." Moreover, she was sad that many correctional officers were going to lose their jobs.

Much like being in a penal rehab labeled WTS women as pathologically dependent selves, the Lodge's avoidance of the criminal justice and welfare systems was an effort to mark social boundaries. Through this process, it could offer "a haven" to its clients and redeem them from the racialized stigma of addiction. This was how Alexa was able to avoid the mark of criminalization, despite the legal realities of her situation: the Lodge labeled her as respectable. While the Lodge was happy to play a role in the disciplinary practices of employers and families, it worked to distance itself and its clients from punishment. Ruth derisively referred to publicly funded programs as "Medicaid mills" and tried to keep women from going to these places for after care. Counselors would sometimes report to legal officials about clients' progress, but they did not see their job as tied in with state governance. Ruth once complained about a probation officer who wanted an opinion on whether a client was "successful." She felt that the officer was asking her to "do his job" for him. It was not her job to decide if the client was "successful" on probation. Success for Ruth meant sobriety, and that was an ongoing process, not a final state that the client did or did not achieve. Ruth refused to make the report. In addition, the staff was extremely critical of how CPS treated women and vigorously supported women in their CPS cases.

The construction of Lodge clients as respectable working people shaped the purpose and scope of its treatment, narrowing the definition of addiction. Its clients did not suffer from pathologically dependent selves, they just had chemical dependency. When I asked Annette how the Lodge helped people transition out of the program, she claimed that they were lucky because they did not get many clients with vocational and social needs—but luck had little to do with it. Instead, the Lodge constructed its clients in a way that rendered these problems separate from addiction and therefore not its responsibility. "Most of the people here are working people, and they're really just going back to their jobs," she noted. Since the Lodge trusted and valued women's families, social networks, and jobs, they saw little reason to intervene in women's selves or relationships in the way WTS did. Moreover, staff members were critical of the treatment methods used in TCs, but only for their clients. In total agreement with the penal state, Don argued that TC clients need to be "habilitated" rather than "rehabilitated." Bill emphasized that, unlike TCs, "we want [Lodge clients] to know they're not total losses." As a result of both the Lodge's racialized construction of addiction and its institutional constraints, the women there were much less stigmatized than those at WTS, and they faced much less intensive control.

That "Might Stop Somebody Normal": The Addict Label and Stigma

When Ruth told one woman that her consequences "might stop somebody normal," she revealed an important part of how the program understood addiction. Addicts are different from other people. Referring to addiction as "insanity" was designed to get clients to see that they were not "normal." The staff saw addiction as a unique ontological state, distinct from nonaddicted people—whom Francine, a counselor, called "normies." Staffers claimed that addicts share particular traits and follow similar life paths, and they frequently discussed their own addictions as examples. They even pointed out how a crazy decision they made before they ever began using revealed that they had always been this kind of person. It was vital that women at the Lodge adopt the addict label to understand themselves and their lives. This had already happened with Susan, a twenty-eight-year-old white drug user who was at the Lodge for three months. I asked her why her situation was different from those of other sheltered young people who go to college and party too much. She said she had been different from the beginning. She described the first time she used drugs, when she snorted her friend's Ritalin: "It was like the doors opened." It was the best thing ever; she never wanted to stop. Susan said that she "knew, I just knew," that she would become an addict.

Several scholars have noted that twelve-step groups rely heavily on narrative techniques to shape members' identities,[14] and the Lodge is no exception. To craft this addict identity, the staff often asked women to go over their history of using and fit these narratives into the Lodge's definition of addiction. In one group meeting, Francine, a lighthearted counselor in her forties, labeled the ten women sitting in the circle with an A or B and paired As with Bs. Each pair sat facing each other and had several minutes to "tell their story" to their partner. But, Francine clarified, not their "whole story." She instructed them to tell the part of their story that directly led to their coming to the Lodge. Afterward, she asked the women to return to the full circle and tell their partner's story. The first couple of women used neutral, nonspecific wording, such as "CPS got involved." It was obvious that they felt awkward describing embarrassing parts of someone else's life. However, Francine then intervened to instruct the women to "capture the insanity" that had led their partner to come there. In response, clients nervously gave more details, such as a woman's husband had called CPS on her, locked her out of the house, and said she was "an unfit mother." Pat, the police officer mentioned above, told the story of nineteen-year-old Dawn, who used heroin. Uncomfortably, Pat described Dawn's feelings of guilt over her habit while she sat at her family's Thanksgiving dinner and her shame for her many broken promises to quit. Finally alone, upstairs during the holiday festivities, Dawn called a friend, promised to go to rehab, and searched for a program online—all while shooting up. Next, Dawn had to tell the story of how Pat's boss put her on a desk job to pressure her to go to rehab without reporting her formally. Each woman listened as another person described things in her life like forgetting to pick up the kids at school, arrests, seizures, contemptuous husbands, failed careers, and profound isolation. The whole experience was visibly hard for many women, who winced with shame. Afterward, Francine asked them what it was like to hear their story told by another person. One woman immediately said that it was awful, another commented that the exercise made it all "feel more real," and a third claimed "it hurts more" to have another person say it.

A-B group taught clients to see themselves as the Lodge's kind of addict. The program mobilized introspective, confessional, and narrative practices that resembled some of those at I saw at WTS but marshaled them for different purposes. These technologies of the self unearthed experiences of degradation and loss and framed them as the result of substance abuse—not of deeper issues in the self. Moreover, these meetings relied on provoking shame but also feelings of identification, camaraderie, and empathy. With a structured narrative and the practice of telling another's story, A–B group constructed the same story for each woman, one in which her drug use caused the "insanity" of her life and "mandated" her to the Lodge. The details of an individual's problems or her psyche were less important than the shared experience of hitting bottom. To be seen as successful, clients must demonstrate skill at understanding their lives this way. Most had been in rehab before and knew how to use recovery lingo. The newcomers, on the other hand, had to be socialized into this new identity. The Lodge's treatment encouraged this identity shift through many of its everyday practices, such as when clients had to introduce themselves by saying, for example, "I'm Susan, and I'm an addict." If a client forgot, a counselor reminded her by asking the existential question, "Who are you?" This incantation became rote for most women, whether they believed it or not, and was sometimes shortened to simply "Hi, Susan, addict."

The ritual of telling one's story was a central technique used to produce the addict identity. Ruth told me this was "practice for AA," whose members do the same thing. These stories, like Marisol's, were expected to fit the standard narrative. Clients began by telling something about their early family life, usually pointing to a few particularly difficult aspects of their past. For instance, Noreen, a white crack cocaine user, anxiously described the physical abuse she had suffered from her father and that her mother had never saved her from it. But these traumas were never the central dynamic. Women then explained in detail how they began using, how it got out of control, and the consequences of that use. It was a narrative of inevitable decline. So as Noreen described her life, she began her recounting of each disaster and each relapse with "sure enough." It was a nerve-wracking experience for many women. Holly, a middle-age black union member and a drinker, nervously told me and Kiley, an outgoing young white drug user, that her story was "not interesting" and she wasn't looking forward to telling it. It'll be a short group, Holly grumbled, about five minutes. "That's what everyone says," Kiley reassured her, but her story is interesting. Holly looked skeptical, and Kiley said, "You sat in your room and drank, right?" Holly nodded, and Kiley mentioned another client like that who had told a good story. Nervous, Holly asked what she should say. Kiley listed growing up and her parents, past, and drinking. Holly said others' stories seem "like a movie. . . . I don't know people [like this]." Kiley disagreed, saying that "we're all here for the same problem."

Moral Treatment

The Lodge is part of the long tradition of treating addiction through moral reform. In fact, many critics of AA and NA condemn their judgmental moralizing.[15] However, the moral aspects of the Lodge's version of addiction actually opened the door to redemption. One day early in my research, we assembled for a meeting of Rock Group, which turned out to be a regular feature of the program. Dana, a white counselor near forty, emptied a child's backpack that was filled with colorfully painted rocks, each with a word on it. Dana declared that these were the women's "character defects." Then correcting herself, because she thought the term was too derogatory, Dana described them as addict behaviors or flaws. The rocks provided women with a list of possible ways to characterize their problem—they defined what an addict feels and does. The words on the rocks included greed, pride, sloth, conceit, vanity, pomposity, shame, guilt, low self-esteem, arrogance, prejudices, hurt, pain, hopelessness, despair, depression, grief, cravings, shakes, power, control, victim, relationships, neglect, lies, secrets, deceit, manipulation, isolating, selfishness, self-pity, hate, anger, and fear. After the rocks were dumped out, Alexa pointed out what was running through my mind: some words, like low self-esteem and arrogance, were contradictory. Dana responded that they are "two sides of the same coin."

Dana then instructed the women to pick the rocks that describe "what you came in here with. When you walked in the door, what were you carrying around with you?" As the rest of us sat on chairs in a circle, each woman took a turn sitting on the floor, picking up rocks, and explaining how each one applied to her. She then put each rock back in the backpack. While this is a limited, moralizing list of problems, it ended up providing a surprisingly flexible rubric for understanding the women's lives.[16] Women could leave rocks with words that they did not feel applied to them. In addition, many clients interpreted the same rock to mean different things. For instance, some picked up the rock labeled "control" because they felt the need to control everything, while others chose it because they felt out of control. The counselors let the clients' varying interpretations stand. Mary, who designed this group activity, told me that its flexibility was intentional. The exercise was a tool for thinking about one's problems. In the end, the Lodge's addict identity was a malleable system for interpreting women's lives.

One consistent element in all of the words is that they are individual traits and behaviors. Even rocks that refer to events, such as being victimized, are phrased as an individual identity—such as "victim." This constructed women's problems as individual moral or psychological failings, decontextualized from their social context—much like at WTS. Yet the list of possible words presented a remarkably different way of understanding the self than was the case at WTS. The Lodge's approach relied heavily on moral language, including most of the seven deadly sins. In keeping with the quasi-religiosity of the twelve steps, the Lodge understood addiction as linked to a series of character defects, especially selfishness. This moral self-evaluation was part of working the steps and was how addicts learn their triggers, assess their progress, and take responsibility for their failings. While certainly judgmental, the moral language had the effect of promising redemption in a way that biomedical theories or TC discourse cannot do.

After each client finished picking up rocks, Dana asked, "How heavy is your bag?" The first couple of times, this question produced a suspenseful moment, but nearly all the women meaningfully said, "pretty heavy." One woman, however, replied "It's kinda heavy." Then, looking like she felt out of place, she glanced around for more rocks to make the bag heavier. She actually wanted more problems! The Lodge managed to produce a desire to fit into the addict model. Dana then asked each woman to explain which of the rocks she had let go of while in treatment. Thus, the group ended by getting women to think about how they had improved while in the program and to feel the bag lighten. This suggests that the Lodge saw treatment as an almost literal unburdening rather than an ongoing personal responsibility. This sentiment was captured by a sign hanging over the living room door that said "Leave It on the Mountain." The Lodge told women that through sobriety they could leave their problems and failings behind.

Women of Substance: Destigmatizing Addiction

Even though the Lodge held that addicts were not normal and morally flawed, it worked hard to destigmatize addiction. This was done in several ways. One was to frame addiction as an alien entity inside the self, not as the whole self. Darin Weinberg found this dynamic in his study of two rehabs, calling it "an other inside."[17] Counselors gave the disease its own agency by regularly describing it as "cunning, baffling, and powerful." In addition, clients watched an antiquated-looking video titled *The Sleeping Tiger*, in which a man in a suit described addiction as a tiger inside you. Illustrated with handmade drawings of an angry-looking tiger coiled up inside a person's belly, the video characterized addiction using scientific-sounding words like "chronic" and "progressive." The tiger is created by using and never goes away. When a person is sober, the tiger goes to sleep, but it can be awakened, more ferocious than ever, if the person uses again. The living room contained a framed picture of a tiger to remind women of this peril. Although the video was hokey, the clients loved it. The Lodge also constructed "an other inside" using a more gendered trope, presenting addiction as a cruel and controlling lover. Women read a "letter" from "your disease" that said things like "I love pretending I'm your friend and lover." A similar "letter" from "your drug of choice" stated: "I HAVE CHOSEN YOU. . . . You'll feel no shame in having gone 'all the way' on our first date. . . . We'll see more and more of each other. . . . You'll soon realize that you've dedicated your life to me. . . . You now have no choice. You cannot live without me and I'll love it! You see, my ultimate goal is to murder you." Clients found this very powerful. For example, it inspired Grace to describe her addiction as like "a bad dude . . . you know at the end he's gonna beat you." This technique allowed women to accept the addict identity but to preserve a valued sense of self.

What is more, being an addict at the Lodge was actually kind of special. Access to the wisdom of the twelve steps and the fellowship it provided made addicts unusually enlightened, possibly even superior to other people. Francine told the clients that she felt "bad for the normies out there, winging it without what we have." Ruth told me multiple times that the world would be a better place if everyone, whether an addict or not, followed the twelve steps. There was a pervasive sense that being an addict, hitting bottom, and recovering made people stronger and better. The Lodge treated its clients as if they were joining an elite club that provided exceptional insight on how to live. Central to this endeavor was fostering fellowship among clients, which helps explain why it was so important to the staff to preserve the program's non-medicalized approach and limited client pool. The frequent use of twelve-step lingo helped create a sense of shared culture and experiences. The Lodge worked to create what sociologists call an in-group to help women manage the burdens of a deviant identity. In-groups armor people against stigma, provide them with a valued social role, and challenge the deviant label that rendered them outsiders.[18]

Counselors' self-disclosures also worked to diminish stigma. Barely a group went by in which a staff member did not talk about her own experiences with addiction and recovery. For instance, even the revered Faye would say "Hi, I'm [Faye], and I'm an alcoholic" before she explained to clients that she ran the facility. Francine often recounted how she convinced herself that she was not an alcoholic because she could bike twenty-six miles. Rayanne empathized with clients' fear of sharing by describing the ridiculous ways she tried to avoid doing her moral inventory. Ruth regaled the women with stories of her barbiturate use, sketchy boyfriends, being a go-go dancer, and having to visit the "clap clinic." These examples show the humor counselors encouraged women to find in the depths of addiction, but counselors also shared very painful aspects of their lives. Sometimes Ruth would take the role of client and tell her story, including describing how she was raped as teenager, got pregnant as a result, and gave her baby up for adoption.[19] I asked clients how they felt about the fact that all of the counselors (except Dana) were former addicts, and they uniformly said they liked it. Alexa told me that she felt that Ruth had a special understanding of her. Meanwhile, Susan felt distance from Dana because she could not understand what it was like to be an addict. In fact, Susan seemed disappointed that her case had been assigned to Dana. This practice of self-disclosure gave the staff members greater legitimacy, but it also made the clients' own lives seem less deviant and promised hope for sobriety. They were united by their membership in this special club—they were fellow sufferers. As a result, there was a relatively egalitarian relationship between staffers and clients that was unlike anything I saw at WTS. Even though some WTS staffers were in recovery too, they actively resented it when clients were too similar to them. I saw the Lodge treat a couple of substance abuse counselors, and staff members never put them down the way people at WTS did with Leena. The Lodge's egalitarianism was possible only because it excluded people who were considered unrespectable and because it did not have the power to punish its clients.

"Thank You for Choosing Gladstone Lodge": Privacy and Power

Gladstone Lodge and WTS both take people away from their daily lives and place them in a well-ordered institution in an attempt to reform them. In this, they share many of the disciplinary techniques that Michel Foucault famously identified as existing across modern institutions, including confinement, examination, surveillance, and confession.[20] Because the Lodge is isolated in a rural area, clients have nothing other than the program in their daily lives. In some ways, this makes it more of a total institution than WTS (although for a shorter time). As at WTS, Lodge clients live on a collective schedule, are required to make their bed, and are counted regularly. There were room checks, and when the staff suspected clients were smoking, there were very dramatic "room tosses" in which bedrooms were searched with much more vigor than usual. The clients clearly felt surveilled. One night when I sat with Susan and Alexa to talk about the program, they shushed me and said the "walls have ears." The Lodge even used practices of collective surveillance and punishment. When someone reported Susan for smoking, she had to read aloud a letter she wrote explaining why she should be allowed to stay, and the other clients got to vote on her fate (although staff really had the final word). Everyone voted for Susan to stay, even the woman who had turned her in. Eventually, staff members canceled the clients' daily walk around the property for three days because of the smoking, which angered the nonsmoking clients but caused no competition among the women. Unlike at WTS, at the Lodge there were no rewards for informing. Lodge counselors could not take disciplinary practices as far as WTS counselors because Lodge clients were actually customers.

One day, I accompanied Mary to meet a prospective client, Jenny, who had just finished a stint in an eating disorder clinic and wanted to learn more about the program. Mary did not make a hard sell. She explained that the Lodge was based on the twelve steps and addressed addiction as a threefold—mental, physical, and spiritual—disease. She also said that the staff members were proud of the women's program and that it was affordable. Jenny seemed knowledgeable and asked whether the Lodge offered specialized things like dialectical behavior therapy. Mary's response was to emphasize the program's focus on the spiritual parts of recovery. A week later, Jenny joined the fellowship. Initially, she had an intake interview much like the one at WTS that asks about substance use, family, sexual history, work experience, arrest history, religion, goals, and so on. Mary then walked Jenny to the women's unit. A white woman in her twenties, Jenny looked nervous when she entered the dining room where clients were hanging out. Mary introduced Jenny, and Ruth asked the women to say their names and their drugs of choice. Then the "Greeter" showed Jenny around and told her the rules. After Jenny's luggage was brought over to the unit, she and Betty went to her modest, shared bedroom, where Betty searched the luggage to look for forbidden items, including alcohol, lighters, books, and cell phones.[21] When I returned the next week, Jenny was leaving. I sat with her in a private spot to talk about her reasons. She said the Lodge was not the right place for her. "They don't do real therapy," she confided, just the twelve steps. Jenny wanted a more cognitive-behavioral approach.

While being labeled an addict inevitably involves some stigma, Jenny did not face a degradation ceremony like Leena. The staff probed Jenny's past and her belongings, but the Lodge had little coercive power over her. In fact, she approached treatment as a consumer good. She could take her business elsewhere if the Lodge was not satisfactory. Other clients approached it as a consumer good, too, even those facing coercion. When Marie, a black union member, complained during one group session that the Lodge looked better "in the brochure" than in reality, Elena, a white CPS client, agreed and added that "the pillows suck" and the women's unit was a "dump." The staff knew this. When Faye spoke to the women she would always say, "Thank you for choosing [Gladstone Lodge]." As Faye chided counselors for not following the mission, she admonished, "We're not giving them their money's worth."

As a result of clients' leverage and respectable status, they did not face sanctions when they resisted the Lodge's narrative of addiction—in contrast to Donisha's situation at WTS. Marie always grinned smugly when she introduced herself, saying "I'm Marie, I'm an alcoholic and a great person." None of the staff members ever responded. Pat was willing to accept the term "alcoholic," but she refused the meanings attached to it. At the beginning of a Rock Group session Pat, who was always a bit of a joker, cracked, "Why don't we just put them all in the bag right now?" Others laughed, and because of this Francine asked Pat to go first. Pat sat on the floor, looked at the rocks, and began to pick them up and put them in the bag with no explanation. Francine corrected her, asking her to talk about them. Pat picked up a few and offered flippant, sarcastic explanations. For instance, she said that she had been told that she drinks because of something with her parents, so she grabbed the rock labeled "neglect." In no time Pat was done. Francine leadingly asked if that was it. Then the other clients suggested more rocks. Pat cheerfully refused nearly all of them. As this went on, the women got more creative and more desperate to convince Pat of her problems. One suggested anger, and then others jumped in to offer ideas about why she might be angry. Nope, Pat said happily. Another suggested relationships. No, drinking didn't hurt her relationships, Pat noted, "because they all drank too." One woman suggested secrets, but Pat refused: "Everyone knew that I drank." Although the whole group tried, Pat was immovable. Later that day, I was with several clients in the dining room area while Pat was trying to fill out her workbook for the fourth and fifth step. She asked for help with some of the questions. People asked about her drinking. Did you hide it? No. Did you feel shame? No. Exasperated, Doris, an approachable white client around sixty, exclaimed, "You're a tough nut to crack!" Clients as well as counselors tried to pressure Pat to say that drinking caused her problems. But she would not, and they eventually gave up. When Pat relapsed, Ruth was happy to have at least ruined her fun.

One consequence of this dynamic was that Lodge clients had a great deal of privacy and control over their treatment. Importantly, staff members allowed them to choose what they focused on during their treatment. Annette claimed that "we want to design the treatment plan around what they feel they need to work on, what their priority is." As a result, confessions were less intensive and never part of a punishment. Like WTS, the Lodge used confessional techniques to shape women's sense of self. All groups worked on a clockwise, turn-taking basis, which obliged each client to speak. Ruth and Mary once realized that clients were trying to avoid speaking, and that the rotation allowed women to avoid sitting next to people who often spoke first so they would not have to go next. Ruth and Mary resolved to make clients switch seats just as a group began to ensure everyone's participation. However, counselors did not confront women individually to shame them or provoke a response. Instead, Ruth told clients that the Lodge could take their money and not do anything. But, she argued, the Lodge was not after money; it actually wanted to help. The implication was that if you wanted to get your money's worth, you might as well participate. Most of the time, confessions focused on women's substance use, relapses, and their consequences. While many clients found this painful, they had a great deal of latitude to avoid mentioning certain things or to use metaphors like "hitting bottom." Quite a few women mentioned that they had left things out of their stories, but I rarely saw counselors ask for more of the painful details. The counselors' interest in getting people to participate without ensuring their full commitment reflected the twelve-step philosophy that if you "bring the body, the mind will follow."

The power relations at the Lodge also translated into space for women to express ambivalence. Near the end of one group, Kelly—a lanky, white, thirty-year-old heroin user—spoke up: "Wait, I have something." She looked upset, and her voice was full of emotion. Kelly said that she was having a really hard time, and that "people [are] bringing me down" by constantly voicing their desire to leave. She urged the complainers to be mindful of how they made others feel. Kelly proceeded to explain that she had just read one of the Gladstone-approved recovery books called *The Lost Years*.[22] Its story of an addict and her mother reminded Kelly of her own life and caused her to feel "lots of guilt and shame" about what she had put her own mother through. Her voice breaking, Kelly professed her love for her mother and said that she realized how hard her addiction was on her mother. In tears and sinking lower in her chair, Kelly confessed that her parents had made funeral plans for her because they were so sure she would die. This pain has caused her to doubt that she could recover, she explained. Referring to her ten other treatment attempts, Kelly asked herself out loud whether she was in rehab "for myself": "Is it just to please my parents? Do I really want it? Why am I doing it?" All the other times, Kelly said, "I was committed but within months was getting high." How she would know if this time her recovery was real?

Francine responded by explaining that being in treatment was like "being in an arena" with "lots of doors." Some of those doors "you may not be ready to go through," but you can open them and "peek a little." You don't have to confront everything right now, Francine consoled Kelly, so be gentle with yourself and go slow. You can go through those doors later, little by little, with your NA sponsor. Francine advised Kelly not to think too much about her guilt now. After Francine's comments, several clients spoke up. Susan said that *The Lost Years* had made her feel really bad, too, but that the best thing Kelly could do for her mother was be in treatment. Others told Kelly that her mother loved her and already felt better because she knew that Kelly was not out on the street. Kelly nodded tearfully. Alexa finished the group with a dramatic and eloquent speech, saying, "You don't have to be totally committed." Admitting her own ambivalence after eight treatment attempts, Alexa asked herself, "Do I really want to be here and do this?" She was not sure that she did or that it would be successful, but she was willing to try. Alexa concluded: "The consequences got bad enough. I was sick of living the way I was living." Everyone, including Francine, was deeply impressed with Alexa's speech. This group ended as they all did with a recitation of AA's and NA's Serenity Prayer, which asks God for "the serenity to accept the things I cannot change."[23] Francine and Rayanne stayed afterward to hug Kelly.

I rarely heard women at WTS express doubts and fears about their commitment to treatment the way Kelly did. Moreover, WTS staff members would have confronted any client who did so about her unwillingness to work on her self. In contrast, Francine told Kelly to avoid thinking about her feelings of guilt. The arena metaphor suggested that Kelly take things slowly. Moreover, Francine allowed Alexa's and Kelly's ambivalence to stand. Because the clients were constructed as chemically dependent, not fundamentally flawed selves, the Lodge did not expect women to be responsible for everything in their lives or to radically remake themselves. The overarching goal was to enable women to return to their life without using drugs—not to create a new self. This privacy and autonomy in treatment is an important sign that the Lodge recognized and reproduced clients' privilege.

CONCLUSION

As the staff of Gladstone Lodge made choices about funding and treatment practices, it also made claims about the nature of addiction. These claims have roots in the twelve-step model, but they depended on racial and class distinctions. At first glance, many aspects of the Lodge's discourse about addiction seem universalizing. The program claimed that all clients had the same disease regardless of the substance they used, and that these women had followed similar paths to get mandated by life. Yet the Lodge staff made important distinctions among addicts. Indeed, I found that addiction was not the same condition at the Lodge as it was at WTS. But this was not because the programs had an abstract disagreement about the science of addiction. It was because the Lodge drew boundaries between its clients and the criminalized, racialized poor. Several staff members argued that the harsher methods of penal rehabs were necessary for that type of addict. Meanwhile, the Lodge maintained that its clients had a different kind of problem, so it governed them differently. The Lodge staff did not invent these distinctions, nor are they simply the product of Faye's and Bill's conservatism, since the more liberal women's staff members used them too. These racial and class distinctions are built into the structure of the treatment field and the penal state.

While the Lodge constructed addiction narrowly for its clients, the stakes of this definition were very high. Like WTS, the Lodge undertook addiction treatment as part of a larger project to respond to inequality by managing personal disorder. For both programs, rehab is not the technical treatment of disease; instead, it is a political, social, and moral endeavor. So the Lodge's distinctions among addicts were integral to its mission of offering a haven to working people threatened with declining social status. The staff and the referring agencies hoped that getting these people on the path of recovery would help to secure their roles in jobs and families. What is more, the Lodge's ability to attract customers—and thus its existence—depends on maintaining the worthiness of the people who come there. While not a penal institution, it was shaped by the punitive turn. As the war on drugs depicted drug users as racialized, menacing others and the penal system developed new modes of treatment, the Lodge staff had to work harder to distinguish its clients and the program itself from this stigma. Still, the Lodge exercised a form of social control that labeled clients with a deviant identity and tried to normalize people to conventional standards. Rehab was not easy for the women there. The program used logics and techniques for governing behavior that are common in many disciplinary institutions, including correctional facilities like WTS. Yet these shared disciplinary techniques did not result in the same treatment. This was because Gladstone Lodge's treatment is not a punishment, and it is not tied into the stigmatizing and coercive power of the penal state. However, for all the staff members' hostility to penal rehab programs, the Lodge required and reproduced the punitive turn's racialization of addiction to offer its clients a way to regain respectability. As the next chapter will show, the strategies the Lodge used to do this hinged on gender as well as on race and class.

CHAPTER 5

Gladstone Lodge

LEARNING TO LIVE SOBER

RUTH, THE DIRECTOR of Gladstone Lodge's women's program, stood in front of the clients for a lecture. She began by asking, "Faith—what does that mean to you?" After a mumbled, half-hearted response from her audience, she continued, "Does anyone have problems with the [idea of a] higher power?" The higher power is referred to repeatedly in the twelve steps and therefore at Gladstone Lodge. Two clients raised their hands. One described disliking the role of religion in her family as a child. Ruth summed up her perspective: "It's what you grew up with." But, she explained, a higher power doesn't have to be that. It could be "nature—the great outdoors." Ruth argued that the clients needed to believe in "something greater than yourself" to combat the selfishness of addiction. There can be no "spiritual connection" if "it's all about us." She then quoted her own sponsor in Narcotics Anonymous (NA): "There is one God and you're not it!" However, a client then asked Ruth how she could "pray to something you can't control." Ruth said, "I'm not telling you what to believe." Still, she endeavored to explain why a higher power was necessary.

Ruth then wrote "FEAR" on the board. It could mean "fuck everything and run," which is the addict's way, or it could mean "face everything and recover." She noted again that addiction "is a very self-centered disease." Then, suddenly, Ruth shifted her framing of the issue and said, "there isn't room for ourselves" in addiction. "Every single woman here would not have treated another human being the way they treated themselves," she said, implying that addiction was self-destructive. Within moments Ruth changed tack again. She described how faith in something greater had changed her own selfishness. I will always be an addict, she argued: "That person will always need to get high. But I'm not that person anymore." In recovery, "I started to do esteemable acts and not want credit for it." Ruth continued, "we set ourselves up by not taking care" of ourselves. Ruth then told the story of a recovering woman whom she admired, who had been homeless and a prostitute but later became an accomplished lawyer because "[she] was willing to do the work." Ruth continued, "we are not used to focusing on ourselves," but being in treatment "is an opportunity to focus on ourselves in a positive way." If addiction was about willpower, then it would be a moral issue, but it's not. It's about putting in the work. Addiction is the "disease of want," she explained. That means "we are never satisfied . . . because we have expectations. Expectations are—" A client interjected to finish Ruth's sentence: "resentments waiting to happen." Ruth nodded. Expectations let others "rent space in [your] head for free," she declared. Ruth ended the lecture by explaining that "we have to empower ourselves," and faith in a higher power is a way to do that because the higher power is something outside yourself. It doesn't have to be "the god you grew up with." "G.O.D." could be the "group of dames" sitting around the clients.

At the end of this lecture, I was flummoxed. Ruth's talk had flowed seamlessly between claiming that addiction made the clients selfish and arguing that it smothered the self. First she had said that addiction was not about willpower or bad morality, but then she had claimed recovery entailed being "willing to do the work" and led to "esteemable" acts. One solution was to put faith in something greater than the self, including other people. The other solution was to focus on the self and expect nothing from others. These contradictions about agency, the self, and dependence were repeated regularly at the Lodge. Mariana Valverde argues that addiction and treatment have always been "important sites upon which the complex dialectic of personal freedom and control/self-control has worked itself out."[1] These tensions appeared at both programs, but the Lodge's racial, class, and gender politics produced an especially contradictory mix. Ruth's first trope was the classic twelve-step notion that addiction is a disease of selfishness yet simultaneously unwilled. Restoring agency over substance use paradoxically requires submitting the will to a higher power, which can be just the fellowship of a "group of dames." In this model, recovery (and thus autonomy) is a freedom from the self that comes from dependence on others and living a moral life. Ruth's other framework suggests that addiction stems from having a weak, dependent, needy self. This is the gendered codependency frame that dominates the approach at Women's Treatment Services (WTS). One client knew it so well that she finished Ruth's sentence. In this framing, women addicts must focus on and take care of themselves. They become autonomous of drugs and other people by being self-fulfilled. As I have shown above, at WTS this logic defines autonomy in an extreme way. It requires that we never expect anything from others. Ruth's lecture not only reveals long-standing debates about addiction and the will, it also reveals broader social tensions over gender that hinge on the value of dependence, individualism, and care work.

Staff members at both programs were attuned to some of the inequities their clients faced. Indeed, addiction served as a way for both programs to navigate gendered constraints. The Lodge's messages to women about gender were ambivalent, much as they are in the larger culture. This chapter examines how the Lodge carried out treatment, why it resisted pathologizing clients, and why it came to different conclusions than WTS about what women need. Although Lodge counselors invoked codependency discourse at times, the twelve-step frame won out. In fact, I regularly heard the counselors remind women that they were selfish. Within this frame, Lodge treatment groups emphasized connection and right living. Staff members did not attempt to habilitate women's selves. There were no makeovers or forced separations from children. The only dependence the Lodge problematized was dependence on drugs. Engaging in habilitative practices would have marked Lodge women with precisely the stigma that staff members were trying to avoid. Therefore, addiction did not signal gendered deviance at the Lodge. Instead, the program taught women a new sober lifestyle based on the twelve steps. This entails continual self-monitoring, with metrics like steps done, meetings attended, and days sober. For the rest of their lives, clients would have to engage in these daily practices to ensure that the risky, sleeping tiger of addiction inside them was controlled. This lifestyle required self-management, but recovery was not a solitary practice. It depended on integration with other people and social institutions. Thus, the Lodge not only worked to give women lifestyle tools, it also tried to entrench women more deeply in social relationships so they could resume their existing roles.

"The Bondage of Self"

The Lodge framed addiction as chemical dependency, so teaching women to live life without using was its priority. Clients must first accept that they cannot manage their lives. This was a central task and explains why the women spent so much time confessing the bad consequences of using. Alcoholics Anonymous (AA) traditionally claims that addicts are deluded and have a false sense of self-control. Consequently, addiction is fueled by the belief that autonomy is possible. This is about more than powerlessness over drugs: addicts have a false sense that they can control life in general. What is more, Ruth framed clients' lack of control as part of the human condition, not just the trait of addicts: "There is one God, and you're not it." Counselors adopted yet another twelve-step phrase to communicate how clients might deal with the limits of autonomy, "Let go and let God." Letting go requires surrendering one's will. Staff members explicitly described this in twelve-step terms as submission. The third step states that members "made a decision to turn our will and our lives over to the care of God *as we understood Him.*"[2] Submission in this context was partly spiritual, but also partly to social norms and to the staff. It also promised clients freedom from chemical dependency. So staff members often reminded women that the world did not work according to their plans but according to God's plan.

Demolishing the belief in autonomy was meant to be liberating. As Francine, a counselor, once said, "The moment we accept the unmanageability is the moment things become more manageable."

In the daily meetings of the Step Group, Lodge clients took turns reading aloud from a booklet Bill, one of the Lodge's cofounders, had written that interpreted each of the twelve steps and gave advice about how to "work" them. His account of the third step acknowledged that "turning your will over" and "God" were difficult concepts for most people to understand. He suggesting thinking of God as a "power that works through people," including the fellowship. Addicts, he says, "are creatures of ego" and don't want to turn their will over to anybody. To challenge this, the booklet critiques the American culture of individualism: "self-sufficiency . . . doesn't really work. Where has the philosophy of self-will gotten us?" When they heard this, a few clients snorted with recognition. Self-will is a "burden" that has led us to dependency, Bill argued. In the end, he paradoxically promised readers that turning their will over made it possible for them to be liberated from their powerlessness over drugs: "Dependence on a program provides independence from alcohol and drugs." In this case, the program is the way of living set out by the twelve steps. Changing one's lifestyle is therefore the path to sobriety. At the Lodge, the way through this maze of dependency, responsibility, and the self was to rely on others, the "group of dames."

Bill's booklet draws directly from AA's most canonical text, which characterizes addiction as "an extreme example of self-will run riot."[3] If nineteenth-century treatments for inebriety viewed the disease as a failure of the will, as discussed in chapter 1 AA suggested that the belief in self-will was actually the problem. Trysh Travis argues that AA's founders rejected modern market culture and the ideals of autonomous, white, middle-class masculinity that should have been "their birthright." In short, they challenged the American ideal of the "self-made man."[4] Bill offers just this kind of critique. Although AA is expressly apolitical, Travis sees AA as doing something radical by rejecting individualism. However, submission has a different political valence when applied to women. In addition, AA appropriates traditional religious notions of virtue and self-sacrifice that often legitimate gender oppression. What might have been a critique of hegemonic norms of masculinity did not decenter men's experiences from defining addiction or engage questions of inequality. Travis shows that women in the recovery field drew on growing skepticism about traditional family and gender norms to challenge this model using codependency.[5] While most of their alternative forms of recovery were not political, some argued that women's subordination and lack of autonomy worked to foster addiction.[6]

The women at the Lodge, both staff members and clients, likewise had to navigate the limits of the twelve-step framework for understanding women's lives. Problems regularly emerged around the issue of submission and dependence. After everyone read a section of Bill's work aloud, the clients had to comment. First up was Cody, a thoughtful white woman of thirty-two and self-declared "crack addict" who had been a Lodge client once before. She took issue with AA's Serenity Prayer, which invokes the higher power. At the end of all Lodge groups (and most of those at WTS, too), people put their arms around each other and recite the prayer: "God grant me the serenity to accept the things I cannot change, the courage to change the things that I can, and the wisdom to know the difference."[7]

Cody explained that she did not say "God" because "I don't know what that means." She was skeptical but "willing to learn," because there are "just a lot of things in life you can't change." Cody added that Bill's idea of turning the will over was hard for her. "As a codependent," she said, "I want to control everything." Submission "makes me very upset." Beth, another client, responded, "I just love the Serenity Prayer." She noted, "My counselor told me to just say it over and over again when I'm anxious." Next, Carla, said, "I did work [when I was] clean to turn my will over to God." But then, she somberly said, "I beat myself up over" not surrendering when she relapsed. Carla explained that the "bondage of self" trapped her, because "I never gave him [my will]." Donna gave addiction its own agency, saying that "when the disease talks to you," it's the "worst thing." It had been hard for her to get older, especially to go through menopause. And so she needed to believe in "something better." Donna added that this was especially "important for women" because "we beat up on ourselves."

This group discussion revolved around the role of the self in creating women's hardships, but the clients ignored the part about selfishness. Instead, they debated the value of submission. Carla shared Bill's sense that self-reliance was a trap. Donna was also sympathetic because she found that things beyond her control made her hard on herself. She hoped that embracing dependence would help women manage gendered burdens. Yet Cody resisted the program's expectation of submission by using the logic of codependency. While she pathologized herself in a different way, codependency enabled her to question the Lodge's encouragement of dependence on others. At the end of the group, Betty, a counselor's aide, reassured the clients that merely coming into treatment was "turning your will over." She implied that surrender would not degrade the self: the clients just had to work the Lodge's program. Like Cody, staff members in the women's unit have misgivings about the gendered implications of AA's rhetoric about selfishness, dependence, and submission. Their

take on these issues, including in their role as counselors, emerged in relation
to the Lodge's broader gender politics.

THE LODGE AS A GENDERED ORGANIZATION

In addition to operating sex-segregated programs, Gladstone Lodge is
gendered in many other ways, most of which disadvantaged women. The
Lodge takes gender separation very seriously. While Faye and Bill share power,
Faye takes the lead in managing the women's program. There were elaborate
procedures to keep men and women clients from seeing each other when
they passed through the other unit's space. Women were often trapped in
their common rooms while the much larger men's fellowship filed by to go
to the gym. In keeping with the classic model of a patriarchal family, the only
men I ever saw in the women's unit were Bill, the Lodge's resident Catholic
priest, and an elderly male kitchen worker who occasionally brought in meals.
Contact with him was forbidden, and we were even asked to leave the room
while he set it up for a meal. During one of my first visits, I unknowingly sat
at a clients' dining table in the men's unit to write up my field notes. As the
men filtered in for lunch, they would not sit at my table or look at me. When
I nodded in greeting, most men looked alarmed and did not respond.

The program's arguments for sex segregation emphasized gender difference, the perils of sexualization, and women's moral vulnerability. These
arguments resemble those used by reformers in nineteenth century to push
for gender-segregated prisons, suggesting that this may be an instance where
correctional techniques crossed over into other institutions. The official reasoning for separating men and women was that sexual interest distracts from
recovery. However, the women's staff and Faye always emphasized to me that
it protected women from the men's objectifying gaze. It also protected women
from themselves. Staff members thought that women have a tendency to shift
from drug addiction to "men addiction." While this logic presumes heterosexuality, counselors did take extra care about room assignments when lesbians
they deemed attractive were in the fellowship. They did not think the lesbian clients would act inappropriately. Instead, counselors worried that certain
attention-seeking straight women would come on to them. "Men addiction"
is apparently a flexible category. Many women liked the single-sex environment, but most of them found the efforts to protect their chastity silly or
offensive. Tropes of gender difference and protecting women shaped the staff
culture, too. Joint meetings of staff from the men's and women's units were
always laden with gendered jokes. For example, Don, the executive director,
once lightheartedly teased Phil, a counselor, for messing something up. He
quipped, "If you ladies would look the other way, I [have an] obscene gesture"
to give Phil.

Gendered norms of propriety were pervasive. In the facility's main entryway stands a sign that asks visitors to dress properly because "this is a treatment
facility." The Lodge has a very conservative and gendered dress code. It forbids
women from wearing shorts on Sundays and from ever wearing sandals, high
heels, short skirts, or more than "modest makeup." Men are, among other
things, expected to be clean-shaven "The message we want to send is one of
confident self-respect," declared the women's client handbook. Faye intended
the dress code to govern heterosexuality and focus clients on recovery. First
and foremost, it was a way to ensure that women did not attract men in
the men's program during their rare chances for visual contact. She told me
this would "protect" the women by ensuring they "focused on themselves."
Faye viewed makeup as a way of "hiding": "You see them [women] come in,
heavy makeup, the earrings, high heels, everything for show. Rather, we get
them down to the nitty-gritty. You're a beautiful person the way you are. You
don't have to add all that cover-up." If WTS encouraged women to dress up,
the Lodge asked women to dress down. For Faye, this signaled that the program was tough: "it's really a test as to are you willing to do anything to get
sober." In contrast, WTS saw its makeovers as a sign of the program's kindness
and gender sensitivity. To maintain a serious, desexualized atmosphere at the
Lodge, Faye pressured the female counselors to wear conservative business
attire. I tried to follow the dress code carefully, but during our interview Faye
critiqued my attempt at a business-casual sweater, saying that "it's form-fitting
and looking really nice, but around here the guys are just—you know." Faye
sought to protect vulnerable femininity, while WTS's Yvonne thought femininity would make women stronger.

These gendered dynamics marginalized the women's program, its staff,
and clients within the Lodge. The practices of spatial segregation symbolically
communicated women's lesser status. When the men wanted to use the shared
facilities, they always seemed to have priority. On September 11, the Lodge
held a memorial mass, which changed the regular schedule of relaxation time
for walks or going to the on-site candy store. In the end, the men's program
received its standard walk, while the women's walk was shortened. Several
women were quite upset, because they valued this time away from staff—
which enabled them to talk freely and sneak cigarettes.[8] In fact, women were
often troubled by the Lodge's gender regime. The September 11 memorial
mass had a complex gender-segregated entrance and seating procedure, leaving the women at the back, on the periphery of the room, while the men sat
in the center in front of the priest and altar. Jill, a white client of about forty-
five, whispered to me, "I feel like a leper." Such feelings were compounded by
the fact that the women's space was decidedly inferior to the men's and less
attractive. After Ruth's "group of dames" lecture, I chatted with a few clients

before lunch. One described the women's unit as "servants' quarters." Another likened it to "giving food out to a stray." All of them felt cooped up in the small space. Referring to what Ruth had just said, one woman joked that the Lodge did this so women would have to "learn about resentments." She was aware that her anger about the inequality could be dismissed as refusing to "accept the things we cannot change."

"As If They Have Any Idea What It's Like": Developing a Politics of Addiction

The women's staff members supported the Lodge's sex separation, but other aspects of the gender arrangements grated on them. They had less power and legitimacy in the organization than the men's staff members, leading to constant friction between the programs. The counselors in the women's program resented their lower status. There were no meeting rooms for staff in the women's unit, so they had to use spaces that informally belonged to the men's program. During my research the weekly case review meetings migrated from the chart room (which housed records for all clients) to two different conference rooms because men's program staff members kept bursting in or claiming the space. When men entered, the women's staffers greeted them with playful yet serious calls of "go away!" They told Mickey, a counselor, that only men in touch with their "feminine side" were permitted. After being told to "go away," Mark, another counselor, entered a few times to do filing. Ignoring the women's repeated requests, he then engaged Annette, the clinical director for both programs, in a long conversation about an article he had read on how to treat highly intelligent addicts. Annette responded minimally to discourage interaction, but he persisted. Mark was finally forced to leave by the counselors hounding him to "go away," which Ruth punctuated with "no gonads!" These were humorous ways of managing the difficult situation of the men's staff belittling the women's staff and women's issues more generally.

During one case review meeting, we heard a male staff member's voice outside the door saying, "It's the girls' club." This outraged Ruth, sparking an impassioned digression to me about how badly the men's staff members treated the women's staffers, including calling them "Brownies." Mary, a senior counselor, was also outraged and informed me that "yes, they called us a Girl Scout troop!" Conversation bubbled up rapidly with indignation, and Ruth gave another example. When Rayanne, a junior counselor, told her story at a luncheon that operates as a staff AA/NA meeting, one man told her, "I admire you for not using while pregnant." Ruth snorted, "As if they have any idea what it's like!" But Jana, an "extended" client who worked as a counselor's assistant, said, "I don't see it that way." She was shocked that Ruth did not think it worse to use while pregnant. Ruth then made the case that the man's comment implied an extra moral judgment of women addicts. This was not something men deal with, she argued, and they don't see their own use as a moral choice but as a disease. Jana angrily disagreed; it *was* morally superior to protect the fetus. Ruth pointed out that the man who made the comment was in the same room with women who had used while pregnant. Mary raised her hand. With confidence, she said she is not proud of doing that, but that's what addiction means. "It was a sideways compliment," Mary concluded. During all this, Rayanne was looking increasingly uncomfortable and finally interjected, "I'm not going to feel guilty for *not* using while pregnant." She asked them to stop talking about it. Ruth apologized and turned back to the case review. In this meeting, the staff discussed gender, addiction, and dependence as it applied to them. Ruth and Mary linked sexist judgments of women addicts with the gender inequality that they experienced as workers. This made it possible for justifiable anger and political critique to exist alongside the language of disease. Through this conversation, the staff developed a social take on women's issues that was largely absent in WTS's focus on the self. So when Ruth told me that the Lodge women did not cook or do dishes (a common client chore in many rehabs), she said with glee, "we make the men do it!"

Treatment discourses typically delegitimate anger and feelings of injustice. They gave staff members few tools to interpret inequality without blaming themselves or their clients. As a result, the women's counselors sometimes had difficulty with the Lodge's traditional twelve-step approach to addiction. I saw this while having lunch with Ruth, Mark, and Ed, a senior staffer, in the staff section of the men's cafeteria. At some point Ruth brought up having post-traumatic stress disorder (PTSD), and half-joked that all addicts have it. Then she lowered her voice to show her seriousness and said, "I was raped." There was no acknowledgment from the others, so she said "I was raped" again and offered another cause for her PTSD, having barely escaped with her life from an apartment fire. I nodded and met her eyes, uncomfortable at the others' lack of response. Then Ed turned to me and aggressively asked if I knew what people used to call PTSD. I could tell he was trying to make a point. I paused, unsure what it was. "Shell shock," I offered. "No," he corrected me, "get off the pity pot." This common AA slogan is used to disparage self-pity. Ruth didn't respond to Ed and just noted that I was correct about shell shock. Ed's public attack on Ruth's framing of her rape as traumatic not only signals the marginalization of the women's program, but it also hints at the problems the women's counselors face when using the Lodge's twelve-step framework to deal with clients' experiences of gender oppression. To compensate, the women's staff members drew on their own experiences and critiques to modify treatment in what they thought was a gender-sensitive way.

The marginalization of the women's program offered some benefits. It enabled counselors to operate largely outside the immediate supervision of

Bill and Faye, and their emphasis on twelve-step orthodoxy. The weekly joint meetings of both programs' senior staff members focused so much on the men's program that Ruth often wondered to me why she attended them. Yet she liked the lack of attention to the women's program. Each day Ruth or Mary attend a shift change meeting devoted to updates about what has happened during the shift that is ending. The meeting is run by a men's staff member or Don. While the men's staffers went into detail, I observed that Ruth and Mary said little in their reports, merely noting things such as "the ladies were good last night." Ruth raised women's unit business only when it posed questions of safety or procedure (such as one failure to search a woman after she had returned from court). Bill and Faye often held the women's program up as a model. However, they seemed to know little about what happened there on a daily basis. Although the women's staff members revered Bill and Faye, they discarded the more conservative features of the founders' gender ideology. I doubt that Faye would have disapproved of much of what the women's staff did, but the program's relative autonomy gave its counselors the flexibility to bring in alternative ideas.

Navigating Gender and Dependence

Lodge counselors are just as embedded in recovery discourse as WTS staff members, and Lodge counselors also turned to codependency to interpret what they saw as women's distinctive needs. They regularly encountered women with difficult relationships, histories of abuse, and problems managing gendered expectations about care work at home. For both staffers and clients, these situations created recurring tensions between autonomy and relying on others, between agency and compulsion, and between lack of control and personal responsibility. Codependency ideas were not dominant, but they regularly appeared as solutions to these gendered problems. When they did, counselors at the Lodge sounded a lot like those at WTS. They agreed with Yvonne: women need gentler treatment than men do. They thought this stemmed both from women's "relational" nature and from social dynamics that uniquely burden women with stigma, care work, and self-denial.

Annette described male clients as "easier." "The pain [men] suffer is the same," she said, but they are more "concrete" about what they must do. In contrast, women are more emotional and agonize over things. She added: "I think they have more to deal with because they are stepping back into the family situation in dealing with children and dealing with housework and dealing with their jobs. I think there's more demands on a woman emotionally when she comes back home than there is for the men." Early in my research, Annette explained why the numbers of clients in the women's program were low. It was late August, and she said women don't enter rehab when their children start school. She lamented how these constraints prevent women from getting treatment. When I asked Ruth about gender-specific needs she said: "Women are complicated. Women are relational. Men are not. So you're dealing with the guilt and the shame. We do not live in a society that says that a woman who has children and family should use drugs and alcohol. It's disgusting, it's shameful, how could you?" Indeed, staffers believed that the Lodge's sex segregation protected women from this stigma because the male clients see the women as "crack whores." Faye agreed, saying that women's issues were "self-empowerment, the self-esteem, the stigma, and learning to find out who they are and what they really want out of life." Even Bill claimed that the world was harder on women addicts. On one occasion when he met with the women, he interrogated Sonia, a client who had a case with the local child protective services (CPS) agency. But in the midst of his aggressive questions, Bill noted that CPS was especially harsh with women and seemed to want to hurt them. He argued that it was "unfair" that there were "never" CPS cases among the men.

Codependency discourse consistently emerged when staff members responded to situations in which family relationships constrained women. During my interview with Ruth, I mentioned Stephanie Covington, an influential proponent of gender-responsive treatment based on the theory that women's addictions stem from relationality and codependence. Ruth interrupted me to say: "She's my idol. . . . I read everything she has and I believe in everything she says. . . . She does great stuff on women . . . being addicted to their partners." Like at WTS, at the Lodge codependency was a feminized form of addiction, and the solution to it was getting in touch with the self. During one group session Jill brought up why she had come to treatment: "My husband beat me up again. I came here for fear. . . . Wow, I wasn't really that strong." Rayanne responded that "we get stronger from within" and suggested that Jill write in her journal about her feelings. When Dana, a counselor, ran a group devoted to codependence, she described it as the "need-to-please disease" and led a discussion about family. Adriana, the schoolteacher in job jeopardy, described the pressure at her job and then her husband's expectation of having a cooked meal when he comes home. Instead, she would "have beer and fall asleep," and "he wasn't too content about that . . . I guess that was a trigger." Yet Mila, a Latina client, said: "For me, maybe I'm in denial, [but] I'm not a people pleaser. . . . I got to do what I got to do." She resisted the lack of agency that codependency assumed, but Dana did not challenge her. Charlotte, a black union client, noted, "I know I'm a people pleaser." She said that she had gotten a tattoo, and "I didn't feel like I had to defend it" to her mother, who was a born-again Christian and judgmental. Dana replied, "That's progress." This sparked agreement from Angela, a white former addiction counselor at a therapeutic community (TC). After Angela became a housewife, she was resentful when her husband would say "Oh, it must be nice [to] do nothing all day." She concluded that "my addiction is perfect for him." Dana responded: "Many times they don't want you to get better. Their whole identity is taking care of things while you fall apart. . . . It's real tough for women."

Questions about care work were especially likely to provoke this framework rather than the twelve-step one. As Faye described it, "a lot of people— when they became mothers, they never really planned it; they just fell into the trap of motherhood." Codependency was the primary response when Holly, a black union client, told her story. She had been afraid that it would be boring, even asking Kiley, another client, for advice. Joan, a counselor, began the group by saying, "Tell us who you are." Holly described having to take care of her siblings from a young age. This was fulfilling but held her back for years. She then recounted the slow beginning of her drinking, which accelerated when she struggled as a single mother. One of Holly's sons is autistic and nonverbal, but she said little about him except that "he's my light." Holly wanted many children, but to her regret she had only three because she suffered numerous, horrific miscarriages. These experiences caused feelings of grief and loneliness, which prompted her heaviest drinking. After hearing about a life built around caring for others, other clients' feedback invariably adopted the codependency frame. For example, Connie said with amazement, "So much pain, so much grief," and commented that "you looked after" everyone. Another added that Holly didn't care for herself, leaving her "hollow." Susan asked, "Who takes care of [Holly]?"

This group always met with the chairs in a circle and a tissue box in the middle. At a few points during her story, Holly cried. Eventually, Elsa, a fellow client, got a tissue and handed it to her. I too wanted to be kind when Holly cried, but I didn't know why no one offered her a tissue. So I was relieved when Elsa did, and later I did the same. After the group, however, Joan reprimanded us: "They need to learn to take care of themselves." Forcing clients to get their own tissues sought to teach this. Yet staffers gave other explanations for this rule. When a new client made the same mistake that Elsa and I had made, Dana explained that giving her the tissue could "stop the process of feeling and expressing." The rule's purpose was flexible, as is the case with many recovery techniques. After hearing Holly's story, it made particular sense to Joan to understand the rule's function as teaching clients to "take care of themselves"—something she felt that Holly in particular needed to learn, because codependency was Joan's primary discursive resource for understanding the politics of care work.

Lodge staff members were critical of gender inequality, but when they adopted the codependency framework, women's selves and behavior became the problem. One day I found the phrases "women more relational orientation" versus "performance orientation" on the living room blackboard. Alexa and Cathy, both clients, told me that a former client had come to speak about women and recovery. She had said that women "think in relationship terms," but "men are more selfish." Cathy concluded that in the men's unit "they do not think of women at all . . . [only] 'I, I, I.'" Alexa explained to me that she had learned that men's attitude was "better for recovery"; women "should be more self-centered." In these moments, treatment became about shedding dependency and relying on the self for fulfillment. For example, after her "group of dames" lecture, Ruth handed out a sheet titled "Letting Go." Unlike the twelve-step narrative of surrender to a higher power, this sheet contained a set of phrases with advice about how to let go of our expectations of others, those resentments waiting to happen. The sheet explained that "to let go is not to care for, but to care about." It "is not to try to change or blame another; it's to make the most of myself." Expecting little from others was supposed to remove triggers for using. In another group session, Ruth offered the same advice for when "we get on that pity pot and we start beating [ourselves] up." This is true "especially with women," who suffer more from guilt and shame than men do. Ruth said that other people encourage women to use, noting that "the people who give invitations to us . . . we have to stop giving them the power." Later, discussing hidden anger, Ruth said that codependent spouses "try to keep you down." She asked rhetorically, "What can I do?" And she answered her own question, "Take care of yourself." This advice suggests women are responsible for perpetuating their own dependence and for "recovering" from it—a view similar to that at WTS. However, the Lodge was not willing or able to carry out the codependency framework in the way WTS did.

Gendered Deviance and Respectable Addiction

Despite the regular appearance of codependency discourse at the Lodge, the women's program relied more on the twelve-step frame. Most importantly, when staff members developed treatment strategies, they consistently chose ones that emphasized staying sober through "working" the twelve steps. Codependency characterizes using, victimization, and family problems as the result of women's flawed selves. In the context of addiction treatment, these stigmas have racial and class connotations that conflict with the Lodge's commitment to its clients' respectability and the counselors' identification with clients. Avoiding the racial, class, and gender stigma of the "crack whore" and her pathological motherhood was essential to the program's identity and the redemption that the staff wanted treatment to offer. The program not only lacked the power to remake the self, but staff never treated addiction as the outgrowth of gender deviance. Thus codependency existed as talk, not as a disciplinary practice.

Take for example Marie, a middle-aged black union client and a lesbian who presented several difficulties for the staff. She not only complained about the program regularly, but she was also resistant. She ate food that made her diabetes worse, declined to pay for her medication, and would lie on the floor of her closet and refuse to come out. Marie was one of twelve children who had the same mother but many fathers, and she had been raised by her grandmother. Marie had a suffered a lot of abuse, including being raped as a child. When one of her sister's boyfriends tried to rape her, she stabbed him. Her case was ripe for the codependency frame and for racial stigma. During a meeting, staff members discussed how to deal with her resistance. Ruth wondered whether Marie had unmedicated bipolar disorder, a form of speculation that Lodge staff did not usually engage in. Ruth also considered whether Marie wanted to be discharged. However, Mary disagreed. She argued that Marie's behaviors were coping strategies that had worked for her. "She never learned another way," but these "survival mechanisms" are not working for her now. This analysis convinced the other staff members, who subsequently focused on how to teach Marie new coping techniques that did not involve drinking or moping in the closet. Although Ruth wondered why Marie's partner put up with this behavior, the conversation did not focus on her trauma or flawed self. Even in cases like this and with black women, the Lodge did not attempt to transform women's gendered selves.

Having read the dress code, I anticipated that modesty and sexual morality would be prominent themes in the Lodge's treatment. Appearance did indeed matter to Faye and Bill, but I found that this concern was not manifested in everyday practices on the women's unit. The unit's independence enabled its staff members to develop a different take on gender presentation. In a marked contrast with WTS, I never heard them discuss a client's appearance at a case review meeting, nor did they encourage women to engage in feminine grooming as a form of therapeutic work on the self. Lodge counselors did not read deeper psychological meanings into clients' gender presentation. The only time I heard a critical comment about a client's appearance was from Judith, who was one of two extended clients who lived at the Lodge for years and became junior staff members. Judith suggested that Susan's dark eye makeup indicated she was not serious about recovery. However, none of the counselors even acknowledged Judith's comment. They did not ignore the dress code, but it was not interpreted therapeutically. I saw clients make efforts to meet some rules, such as not showing their shoulders and covering up facial piercings with bandages. But other rules were regularly flouted, including the requirements to wear loose-fitting clothing, only light makeup, and minimal jewelry. When counselors did mention the dress code to clients, they used nontherapeutic arguments. For instance, Ruth reminded them to wear shoes with backs and low heels so that they would not trip and sue the Lodge. Both clients and staff members mocked the dress code. Clients regularly joked about this attempt to protect their chastity. Dana was dismissive of it when she told me that the fitted suit jacket she regularly wore to work was too short to meet Faye's expectation that it cover her hips. Another time, Francine, a counselor, bounded up to Annette in flip-flops to show off her new foot tattoo. Francine grinned as she showed me that she had tied a ribbon from the flip-flop around her ankle to ensure that it had a back, following the dress code in letter but not in spirit.

The one time that I saw the Lodge address appearance drew on the codependency frame. Ruth cancelled an afternoon therapeutic group to do something more fun. She brought in variously colored chiffon scarves and draped them on each client and me. Based on which colors looked good on us, Ruth then divided us into winters, summers, springs, and falls. We could use these categories (a venerable fashion trick) to choose the clothes and makeup that best matched our bodies. Ruth lectured the group about when she was young and in "active addiction." Back then she didn't even know what colors she liked. This lack of self-knowledge was part of the addiction, but in recovery she was able to develop a sense of self. She explained this by saying that women think relationally, whereas men think about possessions. To combat this feminine relationality, women should learn about themselves. Yet this activity was unusual. Women whom WTS staff members would have chastised for their heavy makeup or tight clothes were not criticized by Lodge staffers. In addition, counselors did not encourage women to engage in feminine grooming as a way to work on the self. So while the dress code gave staffers the ability to police women's appearance, they did not. This reflected the Lodge's presumptions about women's respectability. Their self-presentation was not related to addiction; instead, addiction was about substance abuse. This approach applied to clients of all racial and ethnic backgrounds. Class thus played an important role in constructing addiction. The Lodge's hands-off orientation to appearance was consistent with its broader approach to women's selves and social relationships.

WORKING THE PROGRAM: LEARNING A SOBER LIFESTYLE

Joan asked her colleagues for advice on what she should do with Sonia in her last two weeks at the Lodge. Sonia had had a rocky road in the program. She was resistant and angry, and she had even once shoved Ruth against a wall. A funny and assertive Latina woman from a rural area, Sonia owned a head shop, selling marijuana paraphernalia. Although her husband used and trafficked drugs, he had called CPS on Sonia for her drug use. While under

CPS supervision, Sonia had killed a man in a car accident while her children were in the back seat. CPS then required her to go into treatment for three months, where she waited to see if she would face criminal charges. Sonia was clearly stricken with guilt over killing someone and repeatedly mentioned her recurring nightmares.

Ruth was upset that Bill and Faye let Sonia stay after pushing her and claimed to be skeptical about her prognosis. Joan defended Sonia, saying that "she wants to work her ass off." Ruth snapped, "She needs to live life on life's terms." Ruth added that Sonia had failed treatment before because she repeats her old "behaviors." But Ruth did not specify what these were. Instead, she suggested that Sonia list five self-defeating behaviors and say how she would normally solve them, and then how she planned to solve them in the future. Then Sonia should ask her "peers" for advice. "We all have problems . . . I've personally got ten or twenty [self-defeating behaviors]. She's got five," Ruth said pointedly. Rayanne added, "I see her [saying] 'I'm doing this, I'm doing this,' but I don't see her asking for help." Joan agreed that "her attitude stinks." Ruth thought Sonia's "guilt and shame" made her think she didn't "deserve" help: "She's not using the resources available to her." Getting help from one's peers was "the best part of inpatient [treatment]." Ruth said that they should teach clients, "I'm responsible for getting my needs met." This was "especially true for women." Excited by her own idea, Ruth decided this exercise would help everyone and suggested having a session in which clients would say "what they're struggling with" and the others would make suggestions.

The counselors raised concerns about Sonia that I heard staff members at WTS raise about their clients. She was not working on her self, she needed to live life on life's terms, she had guilt and shame, and she didn't provide for her own needs. Moreover, they knew she had been involved in drug trafficking and that she had killed someone. Yet Ruth did not construct her as a criminal. They knew she was plagued with nightmares. Yet there was little discussion of what her deep issues were. Instead of focusing on Sonia's trauma or disordered self, Ruth's response was to target Sonia's techniques for managing daily life: her "self-defeating behaviors." Ruth also framed this as the kind of problems she herself has, not unusual pathologies. In addition, the staff sought to give her social support. Sonia was not only able to decide what problems to focus on, staff members assumed that she was entitled to help. In short, Sonia had to change how she approached the challenges of everyday life and learn to rely on others.

Instead of remaking women's selves, the Lodge focused on helping them make practical changes to address using and thus enable women to reenter their existing social roles. The program's main treatment technique was to "work" the twelve steps. "Working the program" was the foundation of a new, sober lifestyle. The Lodge asked clients to go straight to an AA or NA meeting after discharge and to attend one meeting a day for ninety days. Doing this would indeed modify women's everyday practices and tie them to networks of sober people. Through this practice, twelve-step groups build a particular kind of addict identity.[9] Working the steps entails daily practices of abstinence, moral self-evaluation, and social connection. In one instance, Betty distributed checklists for the women to use in a nightly "moral inventory," which is part of the continual self-monitoring work required in the steps. One checklist listed the "personality characteristics of self-will" and the "personality characteristics of God's will." The bad personality characteristics included most of the flaws and sins featured in Rock Group (discussed in chapter 4), but the list began with "selfish and self seeking." It also included "self-pity," "self-justification," "self-importance," and "self-condemnation." Betty summed them up as "all about me." The positive characteristics included "honesty," "courage," "grateful," "calm," "tolerance," "interest in others," "good deeds," "self-forgetfulness," and "humility." This kind of daily task seeks to reduce individualism and control what staff saw as addict tendencies, while also promising greater autonomy through measuring and tracking the self.

Rehab at the Lodge operated primarily as training for joining AA or NA. Some techniques were eminently practical. Many trained clients in the cultural skills needed to join twelve-step groups, which have a distinctive lingo and social norms. Regularly saying "I'm [name], and I'm an addict" and telling one's story operate as rehearsals for meetings of NA or AA. In addition to having a daily group meeting on the steps and watching movies about AA's history, Lodge clients heard outside AA members and counselors tell their stories. To help women learn the lingo, they played twelve-step charades. Francine passed around a basket containing small strips of paper, with one of the many AA slogans written on each strip. Everyone, including Francine and me, had to act out a saying while the group guessed what it was. The person who got it right first picked the next performer. Alexa had been in treatment eight times before and was so fluent in the lingo that she often won. Eventually Francine banned her from answering. Alexa's was not a simple skill. The slogans are hard to act out:

SAMPLE SLOGANS

There's nothing that a drink/drug won't make worse.

Poor me, poor me, pour me another.

Keep coming back.

E.G.O. = Easing God Out.

Analysis means paralysis.

Progress not perfection.

Easy does it.

Sick and tired of being sick and tired.

Once an alcoholic or addict, always an alcoholic or addict.

I'm here because I'm not all there.

An attitude of gratitude.

Scholars argue that AA offers social redemption because its narratives of recovery describe past brushes with lower-class deviance followed by current adherence to middle-class norms.[10] In a similar way, the Lodge seeks to shape clients' identities, but it did not try to habilitate women's selves or relationships. Instead, it aimed to reintegrate women into their existing roles through practical techniques of right living. Working the program promised not only sobriety, but also the recovery of respectable social status. A key part of this redemption was to reframe women's existing situations as valuable rather than deviant. In one month I witnessed at least three groups devoted to gratitude. Dana passed around a photocopied sheet called "Simple Abundance,"[11] sections of which the clients took turns reading aloud. It emphasized the value of being grateful for what you already have rather than focusing on what is lacking. It asked clients to write a "gratitude journal" each day, even if they didn't feel grateful, because by showing gratitude we become happier. Then followed a list of 150 "often overlooked blessings," which included taking a nap, pets, and witnessing the birth of a new life. It also included stereotypically feminine things, such as fitting into last year's clothes, taking a warm bath, and having "a dance partner who makes you feel like Ginger Rogers." In the discussion afterward, Noreen, a middle-aged white client, commented with pleasant surprise that she "never thought about being thankful for my animals." Through this process, the Lodge advocated not making major life changes.

The Lodge distinguished between the authentic state of "sobriety" and simply not using, which staff members referred to as being "dry" or "clean." While being clean was essential, staying clean required living a sober life. One exercise taught this distinction. Women took turns reading aloud from a twelve-point list describing sobriety. It meant reacting to everyday challenges with patience, having humility, postponing gratification, "responding to the needs of others," remaining calm, and being dependable. Problematic, unsober reactions like bitterness or selfishness led to using. Ruth asked the women for examples. After one item about how sober people settle disputes without using violence or destruction, Ashley (a young white client) explained that she was angry because her family members were not going to allow her out alone, even to get a haircut. Ruth first assured her that they were merely scared. Ashley then said that her brother was not even going to let her attend NA meetings, and Sarah, the nurse described in chapter 1, exclaimed that this was more important than getting a haircut. Ruth agreed to set up a conference call with Ashley's family to explain the importance of NA. At the end of the session, Ruth read aloud the last item in the list: "sobriety means growing up." Unlike the staffers at WTS, Ruth did not attempt to disengage Ashley from her family, even when they might have impeded sobriety.

The twelve steps famously require followers to admit the wrongs they have committed, but at the Lodge lack of control was not seen as the shameful state it was considered to be at WTS. At the Lodge the rhetoric of letting go did not mean letting go of people; instead, women had to let go of their belief in self-control. Thus the Lodge sought to diminish women's feelings of personal responsibility for their lives. Much as Rock Group framed recovery as unburdening, various other activities reminded clients of the limits of autonomy. Each woman received a small, unfinished wooden box, called a "God Box." Clients decorated their God Boxes during the evening time set aside for crafts. Each woman was supposed to write all her wishes and worries about the future on slips of paper, and put them in her God Box. The goal was to remind the women that the future was in God's hands, not theirs. The sheet explaining the box stated, "If life puts you in a situation you cannot handle, don't attempt to resolve it." Leave the concern in your "something for God to do" box. Staff members believed that this practice freed women to live "one day at a time," with a focus on staying sober. Dana even told one client to wear a rubber band on her wrist and snap it every time she worried about the future. All rehabs must concentrate clients on the treatment process. At WTS, this meant focusing on transforming the dependent self. In contrast, the Lodge focused clients on the task of staying sober by reducing their responsibility to be autonomous. This served as the Lodge's response to gendered obligations, needs, and trauma and protected clients from the stigma of having a dependent self that is addicted to punishment.

Depending on Others: Recovery through Social Integration

At the Lodge, treating addiction meant teaching addicts to depend on others. So in addition to teaching women practical techniques for living sober, the program sought to integrate the women into family, work, and twelve-step groups. This was interpreted as part of the process of "submission" to a "higher power," even if that was a group of dames. Moreover, strengthening the links women had to their existing social relationships was essential to the Lodge's efforts to redeem clients. The women's staff was aware of the constraining effects of gender roles and worried that fraught relationships would distract women from recovery. Ruth once advised clients against calling their family members too often while in treatment. Sometimes the phone was like "1–800–dial–pain," she joked. Yet the staff almost never urged women to distance themselves from their families or romantic partners. Staffers hoped that living sober would enable women to manage strains in these relationships without using. They knew the women had problems, but because the Lodge defined its clients as worthy, it considered their social relationships to be, too.

Relying on the Fellowship

In one staff meeting, Mary brought up Noreen, who would be leaving the Lodge soon and was "very scared" about "picking up" crack again. Mary noted that crack provoked a powerful addiction, and on top of that, Noreen was having trouble with her husband. He had visited the Lodge for counseling sessions, and Mary felt that had been good for Noreen. Still, she wondered if the Lodge could get Noreen's insurance company to pay for a longer stay. Her colleagues decided to look into this, but they were not confident that they would succeed. Instead, Francine suggested linking Noreen up with a Lodge alumna who lived in her area and was still sober. They'd get along, Francine thought, and they could go to NA meetings together. Mary said that this was a great idea and thanked her colleagues for their help. Fellowship with other addicts—in rehab and in NA or AA—mattered deeply to Lodge staff members. Several told me that "the fellowship does 80 percent of the work" of treatment. Counselors frequently assessed the state of the fellowship. A "good" fellowship showed a collective identification, commitment to recovery, and mutual support. When Faye explained the rationale behind sex-segregated treatment, she emphasized fellowship: "We feel that they [clients] need to be empowered by other women. They need to learn how to be part of a team with other women, the sisterhood, the power of the sisterhood." For the Lodge, reliance on other women not only helped clients stay sober, it also challenged their subordination.

The Lodge resembled WTS in its use of peer feedback, storytelling, and group living. The fellowship provided both control and support. The program relied on it to help women through treatment, such as convincing them to stay when they wanted to leave. Jessie's roommates even stayed up night after night caring for her while she went through the difficult process of opiate withdrawal. Meanwhile, women who were suspected of bulimia were given "buddies" who would follow them to the bathroom after meals to ensure that they did not purge. Staff members viewed the inevitable strains of living together as useful tools for training women to deal with interpersonal conflicts. For instance, Cody and Donna, roommates who were both white, had a conflict due to the racist and homophobic things that Donna said. Cody was upset because her brother was black and she had gay friends. In addition,

Donna had taken the better of the two beds without negotiating for it. Cody complained to the staff. Mary was happy when she heard that Cody had "called out" Donna on her bigotry. However, the staff would not allow Cody to switch rooms, because she had something to learn, too. Joan told her that Donna had been "put in your path for a reason—to make you deal with your boundaries." During a session of Rock Group that week, Cody picked up the rock that said "prejudices" and explained why they upset her, but she did not mention Donna. In group sessions, hostile confrontation was not acceptable.

In contrast to the competitive, confrontational confessions documented at penal rehab programs,[12] the Lodge used confessions to build camaraderie among clients through their shared addict identity. Staff members wanted them to feel less alone and less morally reprehensible. In one session, clients stood in a circle, with one of them in the middle—Susan was first. Dana asked her to name one thing she had done "while in active addiction" that she was not proud of. The other clients who had done the same thing had leave their spot and run to an empty one. The person who didn't find a spot was the next to be in the middle. Susan said getting in a car accident. Giggling, the women switched places in a mad, confused dash, leaving Becca in the middle. She said, not knowing how you got home. The next two women's actions were losing a job and getting a DWI (driving while intoxicated). Martha looked embarrassed. No one else will have done what I did, she worried, and she said, "Stealing from your kids." But Sylvia left her spot and was stuck in the middle. Dana smiled at Martha and said, "See, you're not alone." Sylvia said, "Prostituting yourself," and two other women left their spots. Eva was stuck in the middle and blurted out, "Having a sugar daddy." Several women hurried across the circle. As the exercise went on, women laughed more and were quicker to say things they had done. Dana finished by pointing out that they didn't have to feel so alone.

Staff members thought that fellowship helped clients to see themselves through the eyes of others. This could be degrading, but there were no take-downs at the Lodge. Unlike the confrontational and competitive dynamic that WTS often cultivated, the Lodge fostered nonderogatory feedback among clients. Mirror Group, which was a regular activity, was the opposite of TC-style therapy. In this group, women are singled out for compliments, not condemnation. One chair is placed facing a large mirror, and behind the chair are two rows of other chairs. Each client took turns sitting in the single chair, looking at her reflection, while the women behind her each said something nice about her. They praised each other for being strong, kind, sweet, or smart. A few young women were told that they had potential, and many clients were told that they could make it in recovery. Throughout the process, counselors reminded each woman to meet her own eyes in the mirror. This was challenging. Most of them tried to turn around to look at the person speaking, as one typically would in a conversation, but they were corrected. Since recovery was a process of redemption, facing the self required accepting compliments.

Race and the Limits of Fellowship

Despite the counselors' efforts to unite women, the fellowship was riven by tensions that ensured that black women had a harder experience than others at the Lodge. From my observations, the staff applied similar treatment methods to everyone, but the clients were split along race, class, and age lines. Some women were kept at the periphery of the fellowship during everyday life. This group was disproportionately black. Although not the only outsiders, black women rarely belonged to one of the social cliques that developed among the white women based on age and on alcohol versus drug use. There were never more than two black women at the Lodge at any given time during my fieldwork. They always befriended each other and sat together at meals. When there was just one black woman, the social dynamics could be especially alienating. Many cliques came and went during my research, but the segregation of black women at the dining tables was remarkably consistent.

Certain women became the target of unusual hostility, leading to their social exclusion and nasty gossip about them. The staff referred to them as "scapegoats." They were almost always black women who were stigmatized as aggressive, volatile, or "ghetto." Although there were several working-class, urban, Latina women, I did not observe them become scapegoats. A couple of white women who struck others as "crazy" also became scapegoats, but they never suffered the outright antagonism that black women faced. Sylvia was one such scapegoat. A middle-aged black woman who was a crossing guard in job jeopardy, Sylvia had a gravelly voice and an outgoing, opinionated demeanor. She was from the city and had been in a TC treatment program near WTS twenty years earlier. A group of middle-age white women targeted Sylvia for harassment. They made passive-aggressive comments to her and frequently made insulting remarks about her to me and other white clients. They did not invoke race directly. Instead, they used coded language that drew on stereotypes of black women. Martha called Sylvia "the loudmouth." After someone praised Sylvia's singing during karaoke, Martha and Carol laughed about how she was as loud as "fifty men." When Carol complained about the many clients she felt did not do their chores, she invoked racist stereotypes to refer to Sylvia. Carol labeled Sylvia "unwilling" because she had been pushed into treatment by her job, even though many other clients were in the same situation. Carol covered her diatribe with addiction lingo, claiming that Sylvia's "denial" was "sad." Sylvia was aware of their campaign against her. At breakfast one morning, she complained about people blowing their nose at the table because it was "not sanitary." Carol had just blown her nose and started a screaming fight, snapping that if Sylvia had something to say, she should say it to her face.

At that day's staff meeting, Ruth said that Sylvia had become a "scapegoat" and they could not "let it go on." Francine reported that clients had asked for a gripe session to sort out chore and roommate conflicts, but she thought the women really "wanted to roast [Sylvia]." Ruth implied racism when she intensified Francine's assessment by saying that the other women wanted to "lynch her." Ruth firmly stated that the staff had to prevent this session. Although Ruth was white, she had grown up in the same working-class area as Sylvia and was sympathetic: "She's a loud girl from [the neighborhood], like me." Ruth's comments signaled that she saw racism at work, but when I asked about racial patterns in the choice of scapegoats, the staff denied that such patterns existed. Instead, Ruth attributed Sylvia's situation to her psychological profile, saying that "she's a victim"—alluding to Sylvia's past experiences of abuse. With this, Ruth voiced a logic similar to that used at WTS: Sylvia has an addiction to punishment that draws abuse. In short, Ruth turned to the codependency frame. While Ruth was genuinely empathetic, the codependency frame made racism invisible and rendered Sylvia responsible for being harassed. The staff's solution was to "have [Sylvia] tell her story to change their [other clients'] feelings." Ruth hoped that this would promote shared identity, empathy, and identification. In my experience, telling life stories had a mixed record of success. When Marie, another scapegoated black woman, told her very sad story, it did increase other clients' sympathy. The following week, I was shocked to find Marie expressing gratitude for Donna, who had been quite unfriendly to her. Yet telling her story seemed to do little to change Marie's social isolation: she still sat alone at meals.

There were a couple of popular black women, but it was clear to me, if not to the staff, how hard the Lodge was for most of them. As a white woman, I was privy to racist comments from some white clients, since they saw me as one of them. This helped confirm my observation that race shaped the practice of scapegoating. Jessie and Angela, well-to-do white women who became friends, explicitly used race to complain about Charlotte, another scapegoated black woman who was—not surprisingly—quite unhappy in treatment. Jessie and Angela complained to me about Charlotte's arrival because they could no longer jokingly refer to each other as "nigga." They scoffed at Charlotte's claim that it was hard for her as a black woman to be at the almost-all-white Lodge. It was her resulting emotionality that really irritated them. They told me they found Charlotte "scary." Angela speculated that she would "stab someone" and said, "I'm glad I'm leaving [soon]." This was a very consistent aspect of scapegoating. Anger from black women, including criticism of the program, was frequently read by other clients as frightening. White women did not elicit this response when they criticized the program. I was friendly with Marie, Charlotte, and Sylvia. I often sat with them at lunch, and they shared personal feelings with me. However, the racial gap between us was certainly part of why they did not discuss their thoughts on the Lodge's racial dynamics with me.

The client practice of scapegoating was the nastiest expression at the Lodge of how race and class shape constructions of addiction. Yet these constructions framed the Lodge's efforts to rehabilitate its clients' respectability. Its methods could not benefit all women equally. Clients' tensions may have also been affected by class. Jessie and Angela told me that other clients resented them because they were paying for their own treatment, rather than using insurance. Angela believed that she and Jessie received favored treatment, such as getting better rooms—and she was perfectly happy about that. I did not notice this pattern myself because I did not know all clients' payment status or room assignment, but it could have been true. Social divisions in the fellowship were compounded by the way therapeutic discourse made claims of injustice or anger illegitimate. Ultimately, it was the Lodge's own racialized mission that undermined the staff's efforts to create fellowship among women addicts.

Integration with Work

In addition to building fellowship with other women in recovery, the Lodge endeavored to integrate women into work. Staff members could draw on the program's connections with unions and employers during treatment to accomplish this, much as WTS drew on the criminal justice mandate. Lodge counselors worked closely with the union employee assistance programs (EAPs) to manage clients—for example, when they selected a "handsome Hispanic" male union representative who was a "hard ass" about going to AA or NA meetings to drive Marisol home (as discussed in chapter 4). The staff felt that the same man was not a good fit for Marie, and he "was instructed to leave her alone." Representatives of EAPs sat in on some individual counseling sessions, worked with clients' family members, and regularly discussed clients' progress with the counseling staff. The EAPs were involved even when the woman herself did not belong to the union. For example, Nickie's treatment was paid for through her father's union insurance. Her EAP representative, who also happened to be her dad's union buddy, was very involved her treatment. Mary thought Nickie's boyfriend was bad news and suspected that he had acted as a pimp. Mary noted that Nickie was "not going to let of that guy, so I'll work on her toward that." She got Nickie's EAP representative to try to convince her to dump the boyfriend. The Lodge also sought out work-based controls for nonunion clients, such as when Ruth sought to change Susan's mother's belief that Susan should not work.

Employers and unions operated as social control and bolstered the Lodge's limited power over clients. While WTS uses the legal mandate to separate women from outside connections (including those to work) and focus on the self, the Lodge's technique preserves and extends clients' connections to their role as workers and to workplace networks. But just as important, being employed led to redemption. Employment was part of what made Lodge clients morally superior addicts. The only time I saw staff members urge a woman away from her job was in the case of Sonia, who ran a head shop—which the staff thought would involve her with drugs. However, Sonia was not at the Lodge because of job jeopardy. The Lodge could not urge their work-based referrals to focus on themselves before working. Besides, the staff did not think women needed to do this. Being respectable "working people" made the Lodge clients' addiction different. Respectability applied to women's family relationships, too.

Involving the Family and Redeeming Mothers

Reintegrating clients with their families was central to treatment at the Lodge. Clients' families were constructed as worthy, even when the staff saw them as flawed, so returning to family roles signaled redemption and recovery. Instead of distancing women from their families, the Lodge tried to manage families by bringing them into therapy. As with work, this helped staff members govern clients because they could draw on other sources of social control, work with their funders, and align clients with the interests of these institutions. The Lodge offered a weekly Family Program, which it encouraged all immediate family to participate in. During this program, family members can stay overnight at the Lodge. They attend lectures on theories about the disease of addiction, group therapy sessions, and private counseling sessions with the client. During one part of the program, the clients are sent out of the room, and the family members have a meeting in which they are asked to talk about their feelings toward the client. At the meeting I attended, parents, husbands, wives, and girlfriends of both male and female clients spoke about their anger and distrust, the clients' broken promises, and the chaotic home environment. Many said that they were there to support the client, but they would believe he or she was better only when they saw proof. Some said that attending the Lodge was the client's last chance. Amy's husband fumed about the $100,000 she had stolen from him during her addiction. He said he'd agreed to come to the family program, but that did not mean he would take her back. He was so upset that I believed him.

At the same time, the clients were in another room, making a list of the things they had lost because of using. When they returned, they sat in front of their family members and read the list. This confession of regret produced an intense emotional experience. In all but one case, the client ended up in tears. The Family Program first provoked a confession of family members' anger and then affirmed the clients' desire to remain part of the family. Watching a whole sequence of these heartfelt confessions was deeply moving for everyone in the room. A week later Amy, a white client around forty, told me that the Family Program "saved our marriage . . . we are starting over." In addition to this cathartic exercise, Faye described a more confrontational method used with difficult clients. For these cases, the Lodge arranges a private session in which the family members tell the client how they have been affected by her addiction. Faye and Bill explained to me that the "goal is to see themselves how other people see them," thus revealing the ways in which their behavior is a problem. The Lodge's use of family members focuses the client on her effect on other people, not herself.

The Lodge valued clients' families, but staff members could be critical of them. However, in nearly every case when they said that a family member was "the sickest one in that family," as Ruth did about Alexa's mother, they sought to bring these people in for family counseling. Alexa's mother was notorious. Ruth even labeled Alexa and her mother as "codependent." The mother was therefore seen as an especially important target for the Family Program. As was typical of the Lodge, the diagnosis of codependency did not lead Ruth to advocate for Alexa's disengagement from her mother. Faye argued that clients "must heal with their mothers and fathers. . . . We work on the anger right away. The anger is usually [caused by] hurt, because they've been so abused and so put down." However, the solution was to mend these relationships, not end them. In another case, Jessie, who had come all the way from Florida to attend the Lodge, had smoked marijuana with her father. The counselors took this very seriously. Jessie told me that Ruth had demanded that she cut off ties with her father because he enabled her drug use. However, her father had driven her to the Lodge and gotten a hotel room in the area to be able to visit her. Because of their use history, Ruth initially did not permit him to visit. Yet Jessie's family was paying the whole $9,000 cost of the program, and she threatened to leave the Lodge if he couldn't visit. Staff members relented, but they insisted that he had to have a session with Jessie and her counselor. The Lodge often relied on clients' families to pay for their treatment, so the program could not easily force women to dissociate themselves from their relatives. Instead, the Lodge opted to involve family members in treatment and fit women back into their roles.

The Lodge's preference for reintegrating clients with family members was true even for women with abusive husbands. Jill, who had a long history of domestic violence, told me that the counselors discouraged her from leaving her husband and as a general rule recommended that addicts neither end nor begin relationships until they have had one year of sobriety. Faye and Mary corroborated this. Mary noted that they do not encourage women to reenter situations that are dangerous. Yet it was not clear to me how this line was drawn, because I never saw the staff encourage a woman to leave her husband. The idea behind this, Jill explained, was that sobriety was most important. Staff members did not want it jeopardized by instigating other difficult life changes. Because the Lodge defined addiction as substance abuse and as the women's main problem, the counselors urged women back into situations of domestic abuse, despite their concerns about gendered constraints. The solution was to ask abusive husbands to participate the Family Program, whose counseling sessions were thought to address violence. Faye said:

> We address the severity of it to see if it's a domestic violence issue or is it just simply that the husband is reacting to a drunken wife who is very difficult [to] handle. We had one husband [who] used to keep a straitjacket in the closet for when little Daisy would get drunk. He was a sanitation [union] man . . . and he couldn't handle her. She would go for the knives whenever she was drunk and try and kill him. So when you get the stories of the abusive husband, you often have to [go] beyond that, and you have to never believe, totally, your client. Many times our counselors get caught up . . . feeling so bad for the client, and they build up a resentment against the family. That's why we insist the family come in for a session. When you hear the family's side . . . it's all in the eye of the beholder.

When staff members thought there had been abuse, they would inform the referring agency (such as a union) that this could be an issue, thus turning the problem over to them to govern. "It's not our judgment call to call that domestic violence," Faye explained. If they were worried, staff members tried to keep women at the Lodge longer, but "you cannot control" if women go back home. The Lodge was reluctant to stigmatize women's families. Because family life offered clients redemption, it was a valued source of dependence. Staff members therefore sought to "heal" families rather than distance women from them, even though this reinforced women's subordination.

The partners of lesbian women were taken seriously enough to be invited to participate in the Family Program. However, boyfriends were tricky for the staff because they were not always constructed as legitimate "family." This was the case with Nickie, whose father disapproved of her drug-using boyfriend. Yet Kelly's boyfriend was also a drug user. He was in treatment at the Lodge's men's program, and Kelly's family was paying for both of them. When her parents came for the Family Program, the staff debated whether Kelly should be allowed to see her boyfriend (which would violate the no-contact rule). Ruth brought up her parents' payment of his treatment and said "we're not here to break up relationships." Kelly was permitted to see him briefly in a public space and have a joint counseling session with him. Susan's fiancé was in recovery but had once mocked NA meetings during a visit, so Bill was suspicious of him. Nevertheless, he was still invited to the Family Program. The Lodge supported relationships that conformed to nuclear family norms, but more distant ties raised suspicion. For example, there was a "no nieces" rule that was intended to prevent potential dealers from visiting clients.

Only one client's husband was banned during my fieldwork. Cathy's husband came to visit her, and they secretly left the Lodge for a while in his car. When they returned and were confronted by staff members, he became very upset, screamed, cursed, and said he was going to take Cathy away. As Dana reported this incident, she stressed that he was scary, had a crazy look in his eyes, and said he took pills for his anger. The staff debated whether he should be allowed to visit again, which depended on whether he posed a safety threat. Staff members had searched Cathy and did not find any drugs. Although she claimed her husband had taken her out against her will, the staff revoked her "phone privileges" for a few days and had her sign a "contract pledging [to] abide by the rules." Dana said Cathy was "extremely manipulative" and believed that she and her husband had arranged the excursion. One counselor brought up Cathy's history of being in abusive relationships. Cathy did not report abuse during her three months with her husband, but Mary thought that the marriage continued Cathy's history: "it just hasn't escalated to violence yet." Cautious about banning even a difficult husband, the women's staff decided to ask for advice from "management," which meant the senior staff of the men's program. At a general staff meeting, Dana asserted that the husband was truly dangerous, and she wanted him banned. She found support from Mickey, an extraordinarily tough-looking, tattooed, and muscular counselor in the men's unit, who had been present when Cathy and her husband returned to the Lodge. "If I think a guy is scary, he really is," Mickey believably asserted. In the end, Cathy's husband was forbidden to visit her again, and she left "against clinical advice" shortly thereafter.

Unlike at WTS, at the Lodge children were invariably "legitimate" family members, and redeeming women's motherhood was a common theme in groups. Counselors and clients regularly reassured women that addiction did not diminish their status as mothers. I often heard women assure each other they were "good mothers" during group sessions. For example, Grace told Denise that: "You are a good mother. It was always there; the alcohol just got in the way." Staffers frequently defended the legitimacy of women's motherhood, including with CPS. At one meeting, Ruth discussed Grace, an Irish immigrant with a CPS case. Her husband was coming to the Family Program. Ruth called him an "angry miserable person" and said his family had been awful to Grace. He's "her biggest problem," Ruth declared. Grace's husband and in-laws managed to get CPS to ask Grace to voluntarily give up her parental rights in exchange for dropping the case. Mary was livid about this. She missed a staff meeting to stay with Grace while she was on the phone with CPS. Mary told Grace, "Don't sign anything! Don't tell them you'll do anything of the sort. . . . Get your lawyer!" Grace was bitterly amused at having to fight to *keep* her CPS case. I never saw counselors urge women to dissociate themselves from their children. Nor did staff members use the codependency frame to discipline women's relationships with children. A client's relationship with her children was not seen as a symptom of her addiction. Thus, the counselors did not tell Grace to focus on her self rather than her children during her conflict with CPS.

In groups, women often talked of their children; sometimes they even declared that they were getting sober for their kids. Neither staff members nor clients responded by using the codependency frame to suggest that this was a sign of addiction. Elena described how her last relapse had been triggered by her feelings about her son, who was physically disabled and autistic. Elena called herself "codependent" and used this frame to describe how she used her son's problems to justify her drug use, sarcastically saying, "Poor me! Poor me!" Elena claimed that she fixated on him so much that other members of her NA group became annoyed. Everything came to a head after a neighbor recommended that Elena put her son in a large dog cage to play, infuriating Elena. She went to an NA meeting to talk about it, and the leader rolled his eyes. After that, she relapsed. Although Elena constructed these insults as excuses, the clients and counselors made outraged noises on her behalf. Rayanne asked, "Do you see changes in yourself?" Elena said yes. Rayanne affirmed that treatment "works" and then suggested that Elena find a better NA group, perhaps an all-women one. Rayanne thus suggested the problem was with the NA group, not Elena. Despite being given the opportunity, she did not take up Elena's own self-castigation for focusing on her son. In fact, to end the group Rayanne said, "We get very selfish in our addiction." With this, she reaffirmed Elena's desire to care for her child. To defend women from the racialized "crack whore" stigma, the staff had to reassert the legitimacy of their motherhood. Mothering was therefore a main site where clients could find gratitude, selflessness, and redemption.

CONCLUSION

All therapeutic techniques attempt to shape people in some way, aligning individuals with a vision of what is normal. However, Gladstone Lodge differed from WTS in how deep it wanted these changes to go. For WTS, women's barely existing selves needed a complete remaking. But the Lodge's goal was to stop women from using, and to do this, it sought to change women's lifestyles. Its methods trained women in new daily practices that the staff hoped would enable women to manage their lives without using—not to abandon their lives. This process acted on the self by asking women to adopt the addict label and thus accept the limits of self-control. Yet the Lodge did not seek to transform the social roles and gendered relationships that underpinned women's sense of self. In fact, it attempted to reaffirm and redeem these features of women's lives. Staff members thought that relational bonds and new daily practices would replace substance use by offering control, support, and meaning. Through doing this the Lodge gave women "identity resources" that research suggests enable recovery—even in the absence of formal treatment.[13] In contrast, WTS stripped women of the social supports for identity in the name of creating autonomy. My ethnographic research cannot answer the question of whether the Lodge was more effective than WTS at stopping substance use, yet it does reveal how the two programs came to use such different strategies.

The Lodge developed treatment techniques that differed from those at WTS because Lodge staff defined addiction as substance abuse, not as having a dependent self. Although Lodge clients were more privileged than those at WTS, staff members at both programs encountered women with many of the same problems. Counselors had to interpret the meaning of these problems—their meaning was not self-evident. Lodge counselors' interpretations hinged on their belief in their clients' essential respectability and the program's limited power over them. Since they spared their clients from the racial and class stigma of criminalized addicts, they did not pathologize women's selves or relationships. The women's program staff shared WTS's concerns about the gendered inequities women face; however, the Lodge staff arrived at different conclusions about how these were related to addiction and treatment. Through identifying with clients, Lodge staffers developed a more thoroughly social analysis of gender than I saw at WTS and often located women's problems outside the self. It was when they drew on addiction discourse to govern gender-related constraints that Lodge staff members sounded like those at WTS. This tension between their social criticism and codependency discourse was never resolved. Thus, counselors' messages to clients were contradictory. As they alternated between the view that women should find autonomy through self-fulfillment and advocacy of the virtues of dependence, caring for others, and sisterhood, Lodge staff members mirrored larger debates about what women need and the solutions to gender inequality. Like the rest of us, they could not reconcile the competing values of autonomy and interdependence.

When doing the practical work of designing treatment plans, Lodge counselors almost always dropped their critiques of controlling spouses and the extra burden that care work imposed on women. There was little they could do to change these things, especially given the program's financial dependence on the institutions of work and family. At most, the staff could attempt to rehabilitate women from the gendered stigma of addiction. Yet to do this, the Lodge worked to strengthen the power of work and family over women and valorize conformity to social norms. The program constructed clients' social ties as a signal of their status, and as a result, its staff even encouraged women to return to abusive relationships. This is a cost of framing substance use as clients' main problem and of the racial politics of addiction. The Lodge did not stigmatize its clients with racialized tropes of addiction and dependence, but because race and class did not shape the staff's critique of gender inequality, the program systematically excluded black women from the sisterhood. Lodge staff never expected clients to go it alone the way WTS staffers did. They therefore recognized women's right to help. However, this "help" depended on reasserting gendered constraints and reproducing racial and class hierarchies.

Conclusion

GOVERNING THROUGH ADDICTION

GOVERNING THROUGH ADDICTION entails a great deal more than strategies to control substance use. We use rehab to reduce crime, make productive workers, mitigate gender violence, challenge the gendered division of labor, repair relationships, craft good mothers, signify status distinctions, and dispense essential social goods. Indeed, rehab is the go-to solution to mass incarceration, overdose deaths, and welfare recipients who struggle with employment. It may even be trendy, as it was for the Lodge client who wore a shirt stating, "Rehab Is the New Black." We ask addiction treatment to do a lot—especially in the criminal justice system, where it is used to manage social marginality. Consequently, rehab is a window onto larger patterns of power and meaning.

As Women's Treatment Services (WTS) and Gladstone Lodge treat addiction, they must decide what problems women face, what kind of people they should be, and what social and economic relationships they should be embedded in. The political theorist Nancy Fraser described this process as the "politics of need interpretation" and argued that definitions of need are central to understanding and contesting welfare state policies.[1] WTS and the Lodge interpret need within broader systems for regulating social life and must therefore participate in the agendas of these systems, however ambivalent staff members may be. Both the rehabs and these systems use addiction discourse to define need and treatment to produce women as subjects. In this book, I have ethnographically mapped these connections between governance systems and rehab and shown how they shaped each program's definition of addiction and treatment methods. In examining their differences, I found a two-tiered addiction treatment system, bifurcated by race and class and structured by the punitive turn. Moreover, I have shown that gender, race, and class shape constructions of addiction. Yet in looking at the program's similarities, I found a shared language for interpreting the causes and consequences of gender inequality. These patterns shed light on the larger appeal of governing through addiction: it serves as way to manage many forms of dependency in a larger context of social and economic precariousness that makes dependence increasingly problematic. But I have also suggested that there are costs to this process. Through the addiction framework, we continue to dichotomize dependence and independence. By pathologizing dependence, governing through addiction expands the penal state, reproduces inequality, and blames women for gendered subordination.

Punishment, Inequality, and Contemporary Governance

I argue that WTS and the Lodge reveal different modes of governing through addiction. One axis of difference is related to the institutions, populations, and power relationships involved in governance. I found that treatment is delivered through divergent institutional and social pathways that target different groups of people and rely on different forms of social control. This contrast underpins a second axis of difference. It produces two kinds of rehab. In the profligate criminal justice system, treatment is uniquely expansive in its services and duration. In contrast, our tightfisted health-care system produces short stays and minimal services. Finally, a third axis of difference has to do with how individuals' problems are defined and the practical techniques used to manage those problems. These two modes of regulating drug users reveal a broader bifurcation in governance, whereby the poor and racially marginalized are managed through criminalization and exclusion in institutions that are part of the penal state. Even if this form of governance provides services, it is premised on the assumption that marginalized people's selves are the cause of their problems. Because these institutions enact the state's power to punish, they also mark social boundaries. In contrast, more privileged people—including the most stable fractions of the working class—find that mainstream institutions of work, family, and the market regulate their lives. Operating through integration rather than exclusion, this form of governance leverages material need, personal relationships, and social shame to press for conformity and productivity. In the process, it also creates valued social status.

I am not the first to suggest that governance during the punitive turn bifurcated along racial and class lines. In Loïc Wacquant's formulation, prisons and punitive workfare programs manage the racially marginalized poor, with prisons warehousing men and workfare disciplining women into the low-wage labor market.[2] The penal state coexists with strategies of governance that work through other methods, often called neoliberal. The sociologist Nikolas Rose says that these strategies operate by shaping and guiding people's capacity to act on themselves rather than through direct regulation or social provision. Linked to the contemporary cultural veneration of personal fulfillment and individual self-expression, these strategies align such desires with the aims of powerful institutions by prompting us to continually improve ourselves through consuming the right products, managing our feelings, and maximizing our health and productivity. This renders individuals, not social institutions, responsible for their own well-being. Such techniques are premised on the ability of subjects to act autonomously in their own self-interest.[3] At the same time, Rose suggests that another mode of control targets marginalized people who are thought to lack self-governance. These "circuits of exclusion" include techniques to reaffiliate the disorderly by teaching them to regulate themselves so they can be "reinserted into family, work, and consumption."[4] If they do not become self-governing, they are excluded through imprisonment. In a society governed like this, addiction is especially troubling because it undermines the premise that people can regulate themselves. Because rehab straddles class lines and targets failures of self-management, it is a useful site with which to document how these bifurcated processes work.

My evidence also suggests bifurcated governance premised on a distinction between inclusion and exclusion; however, it does not quite fit either Rose's or Wacquant's account. Both WTS and Gladstone Lodge are navigating problems of self-control and self-fulfillment and begin with the premise that their clients cannot manage themselves. In many ways the Lodge resembles dominant theories of neoliberal governance. It sought to enhance women's ability to control and improve the self and assumed their capacity to follow the twelve steps. If they did this, the Lodge promised freedom from dependence on drugs. Women there had to be vigilant to manage the ever-present danger of the addict inside. This required continual self-monitoring through the daily practices of moral self-evaluation and measurement. Yet the Lodge is not a fan of consumerism or individualism. Its clients are not told that consumption is the path to liberty (perhaps aside from the consumption of twelve-step books). Most importantly, Lodge clients were not alone in this process of self-monitoring: they were entitled to help. Indeed, solidarity, not individuation, was a key aim of the program. However, that solidarity excluded the poor and racially marginalized and was premised on gender difference. In this way, the Lodge used addiction to mount a critique of individualism and revalue dependence. It offered women a way to manage the pitfalls of consumerism, individualism, and responsibility. But in its efforts to ensure inclusion, it also upheld hierarchies that excluded racialized others.

WTS, meanwhile, pathologized dependency. With their dependent selves, its clients were also failed citizens. WTS bears the mark of widespread discourses about empowerment, getting in touch with oneself, and self-actualization. Its methods likewise required self-monitoring through the confession of gut-level suffering and identifying pathological patterns. Staff members aimed to create women who could regulate themselves, but this autonomy was premised on their exclusion from state benefits, work, sexuality, and motherhood. Indeed, from the staff's perspective, the women would be autonomous only once they no longer needed any of these things. WTS's treatment, therefore, did not restore citizenship or push women into work. Like the rest of the penal system, it held rights and benefits hostage to women's self-transformation. With its makeovers, the primary inclusion WTS promised was through consumption. Gendered consumerism was both a marker of liberty and the path to self-actualization. Thus, WTS was not about reaffiliation or inclusion. Even the staff's ideal success story—a woman who needed nothing but herself to be happy—assumed that the clients could not be "useful," something the Lodge assumed that its clients were. WTS's model of womanhood and citizenship was premised on social abandonment. This circuit operates through exclusion by criminalizing failures of self-control. Based on the assumption that criminalized women cannot contribute to society, it disentitles women from social assistance and fills that gap with completely autonomous self-fulfillment.[5] In contrast, the Lodge's circuit of inclusion governs failures of individualism through both ongoing self-improvement and increasing interdependence to create useful, productive people.

We cannot understand these two modes of governance without placing them in the context of contemporary punishment. It was the war on drugs that produced the pathways women took to WTS, including policing and sentencing, but also drug testing parolees, the "zero tolerance" to drugs of the city's child protective services (CPS) agency, and the panics over crack babies and pathological welfare queens. WTS's construction of addiction distills the rhetoric of the punitive turn. Because of the program's power to punish, the addict label and the treatment process marked WTS women with a totalizing stigma. Despite WTS's claims to be an alternative to punitive sanctions, its clients do not escape the moral and social condemnation embedded in punishment, including its racialized edge and its fundamental deprivation of freedom. I have shown that the stigma of criminalization and penal power have profound effects on microlevel processes of governance. In framing women's problems as a result of what WTS's executive director called their own addiction to pain and punishment, WTS suggested that the women were responsible for their own suffering and marginalization. By preventing women from deciding their own priorities or retaining their privacy, WTS undermined their attempts to achieve responsible citizenship. In targeting women's codependent relations with lovers, children, and other family members, WTS devalued their motherhood, claimed that their sexuality was destructive, and assumed that their communities were too pathological to save. As a mode of governance, habilitation is organized not only around the idea of addiction, but also through punishment.

Gladstone Lodge also reflects the contemporary politics of punishment, although more obliquely. David Garland argues that structural and cultural changes in the late twentieth century created widespread anxiety and support for a "culture of control," which fueled the punitive turn.[6] It was this culture that underpinned the Lodge's program. There, I witnessed anxieties about middle-class downward mobility, loosening morals, the failure of the state to provide security, and changing racial hierarchies get framed by discourse about crime. Being a rehab program and thus connected to drug use, family disorder, and crime, the Lodge had to work especially hard to distinguish itself and its clients from the specter of racialized, criminal addicts. Not only did it do this organizationally through its funding decisions, but it also made these distinctions symbolically through its construction of addiction and treatment techniques. In their mission to redeem clients and defend their declining social status, Lodge counselors drew on existing twelve-step narratives about hitting bottom and subsequent recovery. These stories all take a similar shape. They begin with addicts falling for the lure of using as a form of rebellion, proceed through their inevitable moral decline and brushes with the "park bench," and end with them renewing their respectability by fulfilling their social responsibilities. Through producing respectable addicts, the Lodge reflects and reproduces the intersecting racial, class, and gender politics of punishment—just like WTS.

The two circuits of governance that I describe are not airtight.[7] Not everyone is black on the penal-welfare side or white on the health-care side. It is also likely that some rehabs serve a wider mix of people than do WTS and the Lodge. In addition, some individuals are able to opt out of criminalization by avoiding penal-welfare institutions. People like Alexa (a Lodge client), who are both middle-class and criminalized, may spend some time in penal institutions like therapeutic communities (TCs) and in the Lodge. Upwardly mobile individuals like Sylvia, a black working-class Lodge client who had once been in a TC, may be able to accomplish something similar. Adriana, a Latina teacher from a small town, used her insurance to pay for treatment at a facility that took Medicaid and had criminal justice contracts, but she was able to flee this "ghetto" institution and switch to the Lodge. It is the interaction of race, class, and criminalization that sends people along one circuit and keeps them there. Thus, Donisha, who was not officially criminally mandated but was under supervision by CPS, ended up at WTS because of her race and class position. The probation system sent Alexa to rehab, but her parents paid for her treatment at the Lodge. Sonia killed someone in a car accident but paid for treatment there, too. This suggests that being processed through penal institutions—not simply having committed a criminal offense—has the power to mark people with the stigma of criminality.

Criminalization is therefore not just a legal status; it is also symbolically conferred by association with punishment. In governing through addiction, the state extends the reach of its penal power beyond traditional sanctions, creating new avenues for criminalization and "race-making."[8] Penal rehab may indeed be the new black. Moreover, punishment's boundary-marking, race-making power is not just about the demographic characteristics of people under penal control, it has racialized our construction of addiction itself. We see this when the stigmatized, criminal version of addiction at WTS was racialized even for white and Latina women. This finding fits with other research showing that racialized offenses (and not just members of racial minorities) receive harsher treatment in the criminal justice system.[9] Racialization matters. We know that "the mark of a criminal record" hurts people's chances at employment, but my research points to other stigmatizing consequences.[10] Punishment marks not only individuals, but also classes of people. Penal discourses about addiction construct a whole population of women as too flawed to participate in work, family, or citizenship. This helps us understand why, despite the good intentions of most WTS counselors, they could never quite keep the punishment out of their treatment. The Lodge's institutional constraints did not enable it to do much for its clients, but it did not punish them.

Advocates of penal treatment, as well as staff members at WTS, value the legal mandate because they believe that it is often the only thing that gets people into treatment and forces compliance. Even Lodge counselors claimed to me that criminalizing drugs is necessary because addicts need legal mandates. Many such advocates also argue that penal rehab can deliver services to the marginalized. If this is done in a gender-sensitive way, they claim that it can help women who have suffered from sexual and domestic violence. WTS staff members shared these high hopes for treatment. Nevertheless, ethnographic studies of penal rehabs uniformly argue that these alternative punishments are not really alternatives.[11] I join this chorus of critics of mandated treatment. Through my comparison of two programs, I add to their arguments evidence showing that penal rehabs operate differently than other types of addiction treatment. Although I compared only two sites, the larger processes that make them different are present throughout the entire treatment field. The referral networks and funding differences that structure WTS and the Lodge shape the field so that penal rehabs have different goals and use different methods and conceptions of addiction. They produce pathways differentiated by race, class, and gender that not only result in stratified rehab programs, but that also create different power relationships between clients and programs. Outside the penal state, people in rehab are customers, and programs must compete to attract them. The discourses about poor, black, and criminalized drug users are pervasive, making it likely that most private-pay facilities will also need to distinguish their customers. Most crucially, I have shown that delivering treatment through punishment comes with a lot of baggage. It brings with it enormous powers of coercion and produces a degraded social status for the client. This happened even though WTS lacked a discourse of retribution and its administrators were critical of racism and sexism. Punishment is different from other forms of governance. Even in therapeutic guise, punishment has the capacity to stigmatize and racialize.

GOVERNING GENDER THROUGH ADDICTION

WTS and Gladstone Lodge nevertheless share a crucial dynamic. Both programs use addiction to understand how gender matters in the lives of the women they treat. They are not unusual in this regard. Governing through addiction is a deeply gendered phenomenon in both its institutional and discursive foundations. The gendered aspects of the punitive turn, from worries over crack babies to the rhetoric of welfare reform, drove the expansion of addiction treatment targeted at women. These patterns even spilled over into the Lodge through the CPS pathway. However, programs specializing in women are more likely to be located in the penal-welfare circuit. Compared to facilities that do not have programming for women, they are more likely to accept Medicaid and offer social services such as housing assistance and HIV counseling.[12] "The largest proportion of women-specific facilities were among residential/therapeutic community programs (approximately 20%)," which is the kind of treatment found primarily in penal rehabs.[13] The gendered aspects of addiction treatment—both at WTS and the Lodge—therefore intersect with race and class. When I began my research, I was interested in exactly how this intersectionality shaped the way women's deviance is constructed and controlled. I was surprised to find that it was the Lodge that urged selflessness, and WTS that urged women to be more selfish. To understand this difference, we must understand the politics of dependency.

For women, drug use and criminal behavior not only violate the law, they represent a breach of gender norms. This fact has typically made women who use drugs seem even more deviant than men who use. When Lodge staffers Mary and Ruth were outraged that a male counselor complimented their colleague Rayanne for not using while she was pregnant, they were responding to exactly this gendered stigma. When WTS staff members worried about the body image of clients like Belinda, they were also navigating the relationship between addiction and gender norms, although less overtly. In 1997, the criminologist Lisa Maher argued that we tend to use the simplistic dichotomy of victimization or volition to depict women involved with drugs. Some depictions frame women as agents in command of their own destinies, opportunistically pursuing their own pleasure or power. In one volition narrative, the decline of traditional gender roles opened up opportunities for women to be as bad as men. In another, women's using and dealing are signs of resistance to patriarchy. Portrayals of victimization, in contrast, frame women's drug use as a result of bad men, a method of coping with the patriarchy, or enslavement by the substance itself.[14] While victimization narratives are often framed as critiques of subordination, they also attempt to realign women drug users with stereotypes of women as passive, pure, and vulnerable. The notion of addiction is key to most victimization narratives. Instead of seeking pleasure for its own sake, such women are seen as disordered and weak. Maher critiques the volition-victimization dichotomy for simplifying the relationship between constraint and agency. Her research on poor women drug users showed that they were simultaneously victimized by male domination while also resisting men's power and innovating clever ways to navigate the constraints of race, class, and gender. Despite evidence like this, governing through addiction remains caught in the same gendered tension between agency and dependence.

The victimization framework dominated WTS and was a theme at the Lodge as well. Yet my research suggests that there have been some recent changes to the victimization narrative. Both WTS and the Lodge relied on codependency discourse to define addiction. In it, women drug users suffer from having emotionally and psychologically dependent selves—selves that are so weak, they do not even exist. Using drugs is merely one feature of a much broader dependence on external sources for fulfillment. For a concept that originated in feminized self-help literature that is associated with often-mocked ideas like the inner child, the codependency frame has a remarkable appeal for the criminal justice system. Research suggests that it is commonly used in penal institutions. In Lynne Haney's study of a gender-sensitive penal rehab with an ideology similar to WTS's, she argues that this narrative led the program to govern desire by targeting how women find pleasure. Instead of relying on drugs, men, and the street lifestyle, women were to get in touch with themselves and publicly confess their trauma. Haney found that this differed from the dependency discourse common in the mid-1990s, which emphasized women's economic reliance on the state.[15] Jill McCorkel found an early version of this discourse in a prison rehab program. It blamed women's disordered, failed selves for their problems, but it lacked the focus on emotional autonomy found in later studies, including this one. McCorkel showed that welfare reform's dependency discourse and racialized depictions of women criminals merged into this narrative of gendered addiction.[16] These ideas are manifested in several related tropes. Sometimes women are diagnosed with weak ego boundaries and pushed to individuate themselves by avoiding relationships and controlling their emotions. At other times, women's problems are attributed to their low self-esteem.[17] This results in the odd situation in which, as I noted chapter 3 the state is punishing women in order to make them love themselves.

I argue that codependency is appealing to WTS, the criminal justice system, and occasionally to the Lodge for a few reasons. Like previous victimization narratives, it is aligned with gender stereotypes, including by denying that women seek pleasure and instead constructing women's drug use as an outgrowth of dependency. For counselors and reformers, this makes it possible for programs to seem as if they challenge stigma by restoring women to an acceptable form of femininity. What is new is that it makes women's selves the agent of their own victimization. Paradoxically, codependency maintains the basic form of a victimization narrative, while also invoking the personal responsibility of volition narratives. This means that it fits quite well into the contemporary penal system. It retains the core of moral condemnation and blame that is an essential part of punishment's stigmatizing function. Linking codependency to criminalization works to re-racialize victimization narratives, which were previously applied more to white women. I found that it was deployed more at WTS than at the Lodge, and thus more to poor and black women than to white or middle-class ones. The codependency frame thus has an affinity with "controlling images" of black women as dependent welfare queens who head pathological families.[18]

Codependency has another important appeal as a governing strategy. Counselors at WTS and the Lodge use it to conceptualize women's victimization, obligations to perform care work, and male-dominated relationships. Both programs linked the problems that women drug users confront to gendered inequities facing women in general. Codependency was therefore a way of understanding and responding to women's subordination. Despite my critiques of these programs, I believe that the women working in them want to help their clients. Moreover, they are critical of prevailing gender arrangements. Codependency was the main discursive resource that they had to manage women in line with their gender politics, especially at WTS. It is telling that this is their go-to narrative. Indeed, the counselors I studied are not the only ones who conceptualize oppression primarily in psychological terms. They are part of larger trends to see disempowerment as a matter of self-esteem and to think of the wounds of sexism (and racism) in terms of trauma.[19] These ideas stem partly from feminized recovery discourse, and their pervasiveness in rehab programs and beyond signals that we are increasingly governing gender inequality through addiction.

As the counselors at the Lodge and WTS go about their work, they must deal with questions about women's role in the family, including their obligations as mothers, daughters, wives, and girlfriends. They meet women who are struggling to balance these obligations with paid employment, who have child care problems, and who must make related decisions about what they really want in life. Staff members also regularly confront situations of abuse, usually from the men closest to their clients. Indeed, the institutions that send women to treatment and fund it expect rehabs to manage these problems. This is especially obvious at WTS, but even the Lodge, with its obligation to its clients' employers and families, cannot help but be implicated in such matters. This is incredibly hard work. Counselors come up against long-standing problems that feminist theory suggests are at the crux of gender inequality: the division of labor between men and women, the devaluation of women's work and femininity, the exploitation of women's sexuality, and notions of citizenship premised on an autonomous subject. All these processes involve matters of dependence. As gender relations altered dramatically in the past fifty years, women's legal, economic, and social dependence has become problematic. Most successful challenges to women's subordination were intended to enable them to become more like stereotypical men—independent. This situation continues to produce difficult binds for women, such as when they work for pay but still have a "second shift" of care work at home.[20] What happens when women fail as mothers, workers, wives, or citizens? We pathologize their dependence. The rehabs in this study used addiction to understand the gendered limits and failures of individualism. Thus, the codependency frame appealed to staff members because they must help women navigate the impossible and gendered standards of complete autonomy.

Yet here is where WTS and the Lodge differ again. On the one hand, WTS counselors adopted this framing wholeheartedly. In large part this was because it aligned with their role as a punishment, and it fit with racialized stereotypes. The counselors attributed nearly all of women's problems to their dependent selves. Making women work on the self was a way to create a new, more autonomous subject. Since staff members did not think their clients really had a self yet, this was an enormously ambitious project, and it depended on WTS's long treatment times and coercive power. The project made treatment very intense. The clients had to work on the self through introspection and confession, especially about painful gendered parts of their lives. By discovering their past pathologies and expressing their feelings, women were supposed to get in touch with who they really were and craft a new self-concept around this disordered dependency. This process also entailed being called out and "pulled up" by fellow clients and counselors, who were said to be able to see a woman's true addict self, which she concealed from herself. Women also had to separate themselves from their previous identities—including being a mother, being tough, and being career oriented—because they were a sign of dependence. WTS counselors thought that this would break the cycle whereby women needed outside sources of validation and sought out pain and punishment because of their low self-esteem. Staff members viewed separating from others partly as a technique to work on the self in rehab, but it was also a larger life goal. They wanted women to learn to neither need nor to expect anything from outside themselves. WTS's successful client does not quite fit the image of masculine independence based on paid labor. She is not the middle-class woman who has it all. Instead, WTS envisioned a new kind of femininity based on psychological and relational autonomy. This was codependency's other appeal. The successful client is a woman who can emotionally endure social abandonment. WTS staff members are correct that this is what their clients face.

On the other hand, Gladstone Lodge was much more ambivalent when dealing with the gendered limits of individualism. In making treatment decisions, its staff members had to ask what women's lives should look like and what they need to get there. Like society as a whole, they were not sure of the answers. Staff members repeatedly flip-flopped. At one moment, I would hear about the twelve-step strategy of challenging individualism through surrender, conformity, and camaraderie, and that the only dependence that is bad is dependence on drugs. At the next moment, the topic would be the codependency frame, in which women become autonomous by having no expectations and all forms of dependence are a problem. Lodge counselors frequently adopted codependency language when women felt constrained by care work or had suffered abuse. But this idea was mostly women-centered window dressing for the Lodge's core mission of producing sobriety and respectability. The program offered women a solution that was both moral and social. When clients spent time going over all the bad consequences of using, the program taught them that they had committed moral wrongs. Notably, this moral language was less stigmatizing than the codependency discourse was at WTS. Similarly, Lodge clients learned to see themselves as addicts and alcoholics, yet this identity offered them salvation through a community of fellow sufferers. Codependency discourse did not inform crucial decisions about women's relationships or diagnoses of their problems. Thus, the Lodge pathologized only chemical dependency and let other possible dependencies off the hook. Ultimately, staff members were unwilling to stigmatize women's selves or their families. Fully deploying the codependency framework would have racialized their clients' addictions and undermined their respectability. What is more, such an approach would not go over well with the employee assistance programs (EAPs), unions, and family members who want rehab to return women to their existing roles.

One other factor worked against codependency: Lodge counselors had, at times, a social analysis of women's problems. When they complained that women's mothering obligations or gendered stigma prevented women from accessing treatment, staff members pointed to social structures and cultural norms, problems that were outside the self. In addition, through their praise of fellowship among women, staff members recognized the value of social support and advocated a kind of feminist solidarity. Although WTS's website includes statistics about how racism, poverty, and gender violence affect the lives of criminalized women, this perspective did not come through during the program's treatment. I struggled to understand why the Lodge staff members were able to see the social forces that shaped women's lives while WTS staff members apparently were not.

One of this book's central arguments has been that our addiction frameworks individualize social inequality, ultimately blaming women—especially those who are poor and nonwhite—for their own oppression. Over and over again, I saw the social disappear in favor of personal pathology.[21] When WTS dismissed Belinda's crises with her son as a projection of her body image issues, they made invisible the structural barriers of poverty, ethnicity, gendered labor, and failing education systems. When Lodge counselors asked clients like Holly and Adriana, whose lives had been curtailed by care work, "who takes care of you?," the answer was supposed to be that each woman should take care of herself. This renders them responsible for managing gendered expectations and inflexible work structures. The very premise of governing through addiction rests on this individualization. The Lodge fell victim to this much of the time through its focus on substance use and moral flaws. Individualization there meant that following a twelve-step lifestyle was the solution, even if a client had an abusive marriage. At WTS, individualization went much deeper, which entailed more stigma and legitimated exclusion. I think what enabled Lodge staff members to see glimpses of social dynamics through the fog of addiction discourse was that, in contrast to the situation at WTS, they had a less hierarchical relationship with clients and identified with them as fellow addicts. For that reason, Lodge staff members were able to see their clients' struggles and their struggles as linked. At WTS, some counselors also had backgrounds similar to those of the clients, which suggests that their role in punishment inhibited identification with the clients. Nevertheless, the Lodge's solidarity and view of social constraints had its limits—as scapegoated clients like Sylvia and Charlotte knew. Without an acknowledgment of the constraints of race and class, the Lodge's already tenuous social analysis of gender could not benefit black clients as much as white ones.

What I observed at WTS and the Lodge reveals the limits of using addiction discourse to understand and manage gender inequality. The counselors in both programs, like the people who created models of gender-responsive treatment, have high hopes for rehab, but the very framework of addiction undermines their efforts. One problem is that gendered addiction discourse lacks an intersectional perspective, one that considers gender in relation to class and race. However, by locating the problem in women's flawed selves, the addiction framework cannot be intersectional. Both programs' treatment approaches made social forces invisible or blamed their clients for the effects of these forces. In the process they reinforced inequality—WTS by stigmatizing and excluding women from social life, and the Lodge by reinforcing women's existing position in the name of redeeming respectability. There are especially high costs to individualization for poor, African American, and criminalized women. Not only do these axes of inequality add additional constraints, but they also interact with gender ideologies, transforming the women's addictions into a uniquely depraved master status that defines their entire selves. By reinforcing the victimization-volition dichotomy, addiction replicates the pathologization of dependency. This both reaffirms essentialist ideas about women's nature and essentializes racist stereotypes about black women and black families. Because codependency pathologizes women's dependency and posits such a radical version of autonomy as the solution, it cannot challenge women's subordination. Asking women to stop needing others or caring for others will not end an unfair division of labor or enable them to navigate conflicts between work and family. It is true that oppression and abuse cause deep, personal wounds. Yet I maintain that the trauma framework, especially without a broader social critique, only obscures the reality of women's lives.

RETHINKING REHAB

When I present the results of this research, I am often asked how we can make treatment better. I am reluctant to answer this question for two reasons. One is that, as I have indicated above, I am skeptical that we can understand or address social problems through an addiction framework. I am not arguing that people do not have problems with substance use, need therapy, or have not experienced trauma. I am not suggesting that women lack gender-specific needs. There are certainly many individuals whose lives are damaged or cut short because of substance use. Many people experience their desire to use drugs and their drug-seeking behavior as unwilled, out of their control. So in critiquing rehab, I am not arguing that there should be no help for these people. However, I am telling a cautionary tale about the way we manage substance use and the work that we ask the idea of addiction to do.

The other source of my reluctance is that my study did not examine the effects of these programs on women's lives after treatment. Most of the time questions about improving treatment are answered by looking at relapse and recidivism rates. Based on my data, I cannot say which program is better from this perspective. Proposals for more effective drug treatment are like a broken record. Scholars have identified the same problems with our system for decades.[22] They have found that treatment does not prevent the majority of individuals from relapsing. They attribute this to the rehab field's resistance to scientific knowledge, its cult-like devotion to the twelve steps, and its poorly educated counselors. They suggest increasing the use of biomedical approaches involving pharmaceutical treatments, greater access to maintenance drugs like Suboxone, the expansion of criminal mandates, integrating treatment with mainstream medicine, or any number of other things. But I argue that by focusing on efficacy as measured by relapse, these critics miss the many things we try to do by governing through addiction. The many goals of rehab may be part of why these programs seem so ineffective. Rehabs are trying to do more than regulate substance use. Moreover, it is possible that the women who came through WTS and the Lodge relapsed but were still able to use aspects of their treatment to help them manage life or find happiness. Perhaps relapse rates are not the best measure of a rehab program's success. Perhaps stopping drug use is not the most important goal.

Despite these misgivings, my research suggests some ideas about what could make treatment better, especially regarding what happens in rehab and how it is organized. There are, however, large structural barriers to change. One is simply the extent to which we govern through addiction. Its practices and ideologies are embedded in many institutional processes. It is not possible to change rehabs or counselor training without changing the imperatives that these systemic processes place on programs. For instance, many people are surprised by the low educational requirements for counselors and the fact that many if not most (there is no way to tell) of them enter the field as a result of their own recovery. This second facet of rehab is an old tradition in treatment and fostered by the twelve steps' demand that followers spread the gospel to other addicts. I have argued that gendered and racialized ideologies about addiction are a problem, but I do not think that they could be addressed by requiring counselors to have master's degrees in social work, for example. Addiction discourse is deeply embedded throughout our culture and serves the interests not only of staff members but also of the institutions that govern through addiction. Moreover, they are not separable from larger cultural tensions about dependency, gender, race, crime, and respectability. Finally, these discussions about improving rehab usually take place without input from the targets of treatment. Indeed, clients in treatment programs have little say in how their problems or needs are defined. This is especially true in penal rehabs. In most programs, clients' complaints are dismissed with "that's your disease talking," and their relapses are always attributed to their own failures. We should start to look for solutions by asking clients to suggest some.

Given all this, I would still recommend disentangling treatment from punishment as much as possible. Because of the stigmatizing and coercive nature of punishment, I doubt that people can get dignified, nonoppressive treatment in the criminal justice system. In saying this, I am aware that rehab is our primary solution to mass incarceration, and I fear that my critique of penal treatment will damage efforts to end this extraordinary injustice. So in challenging penal addiction treatment, I am not arguing for mere incarceration instead. But removing the penal system from rehab should not mean creating more programs like WTS, which are private agencies. They still carry out the state's power to punish. Separating the penal system and rehab requires fundamental changes to both punishment and the provision of welfare services. It certainly means punishing fewer people and limiting or ending the criminalization of drug use. But it is not clear what this would look like institutionally for rehab programs. Making sentences and parole decisions less dependent on clients' therapeutic progress would help make this separation possible. It is important to give poor and criminalized people the same access to privacy that more privileged folks expect from their therapists—something WTS women never had. It is impossible to deal in meaningful and humane ways with devastating issues like trauma when prison is hanging over your head. Penal rehabs like WTS are not safe spaces for therapeutic work. Likewise, the system should abandon its preference for the TC method, which is the source of many of the harshest aspects of penal rehabs. Nevertheless, as I have shown, it is impossible to avoid punishment's power to stigmatize, even at comprehensive alternative programs like WTS. Distancing treatment from punishment also means disentangling it from access to social welfare services. People should not have to be criminalized to get treatment or other social services. Advocates of penal rehabs argue that they are great places to deliver services to the poor, and there certainly are lots of poor people in them. But we should not make access to social citizenship contingent on criminalization.

Although criminalizing drug use has had terrible social consequences, merely turning drug users over to the health-care system is also problematic. If we eliminated penal-welfare funding for rehab programs, the poor would have limited access to treatment, even with health-care reforms such as the Affordable Care Act. Moreover, eliminating penal funding alone will not also eliminate the consequences of racial and class stigma. Nevertheless, I agree with the Gladstone Lodge staff that insurance companies should cover more and longer treatment. We should also support a wider range of treatment approaches. The emphasis on abstinence-only treatment is embedded in recovery culture and penal mandates. This fuels the dominance of twelve-step methods, which have a place in treatment but cannot be the only method aside from penal TCs. The emphasis on abstinence distorts treatment's larger aim to improve lives. I therefore support harm reduction measures that do not require abstinence and instead seek to reduce the risks of substance use.

Most fundamentally, I argue for abandoning the belief that addiction can explain social problems and that rehab can address them. WTS's expansive version of addiction imparted stigma and legitimated punitive forms of control that the addict label did not at Gladstone Lodge. Yet the staff of both programs were unable to tackle the hardships in women's lives and participated in excluding the marginalized. By revealing addiction to be a racialized, gendered, and class-based category, I have shown that governing through addiction repro-duces inequality. Changing this process requires bringing social dynamics back into our frameworks for understanding poverty, gender subordination, and racial marginalization. For addiction treatment to help people, it cannot be the only governing logic in play. If rehabs continue to deliver social services, then we must enable counselors to see their work through other lenses. The individualization of addiction frameworks is exacerbated by counselors' low pay and poor working conditions. Throughout this book, I have been critical of their actions, but they do very difficult work. As we govern through addic-tion, we place the hardest, most complex social problems in their hands. Ulti-mately, I think the solution is to not expect rehab to do that much. We must turn elsewhere for solutions. This entails changing dominant narratives about gender, race, and dependency and instituting more substantive social changes. In governing through addiction, the programs I studied cut off social and political critique. They made women's anger pathological and their expecta-tions of people and institutions disordered. In short, it disempowered them. The women at the Lodge could perhaps find solace in fellowship with other women. But for the women at WTS, the addiction framework only enforced their exclusion by enabling their social abandonment. It is not the women at WTS who are addicted to punishment, it is the society around them.

METHODOLOGICAL APPENDIX

LIKE MOST studies, especially ethnographic ones, mine was not a linear process. I began with a set of theoretical and empirical questions, and these questions evolved over the course of my research as I expanded an analysis of Women's Treatment Services (WTS) into a comparative study of it and Gladstone Lodge. This project draws on the extended case method of ethnography outlined by Michael Burawoy.[1] I was therefore guided by a theoretical orientation and looked for ethnographic sites that enabled me to use microlevel data about a particular context to refine existing theories of larger-scale processes. Because my sites differed from each other in systematic ways, I was able to reveal how larger structural and cultural forces impinged on everyday practice. The comparison was strategic, with the goal of "extending out" to theory rather than using quantitative notions of generalizability, which are especially difficult to apply (nor always desirable) in ethnographic research.[2] Since sociological theories are invariably inadequate for grasping the complexity of social life, the extended case method aims to place theoretical accounts in dialogue with those of the people we study and connect micro to macro. Surprising or anomalous ethnographic evidence then helps rework theory. Ethnographic research is particularly important for this process because surveys and interviews cannot get at practices or interactions among people and how these are affected by their relationships with larger structures. Indeed, if I had only interviewed staff members, the stock narratives of recovery culture would have made WTS and the Lodge look more similar than I found them to be.[3] Power relations shaped the process of site selection and ethnographic research in ways that affected my findings. But by attending to these power dynamics, I found them to be revealing sources of information about the treatment field and the relationships between staff members and clients.

SITE SELECTION AND ENTRY

I first came to WTS as a volunteer while I was in graduate school and wondered if it would make a good research site. Spurred by feminist scholarship about the intersecting racial and gender politics that shape state approaches to mothers who use drugs, I wanted to examine how penal institutions construct the women they manage and how state governance shapes the regulation of gender deviance. In particular, I was looking for a case where I could see how this process played out in the context in which extreme punitiveness coexisted with emerging forms of community-based punishment carried out by private actors. I found WTS via its website, which was unusually snazzy for a penal rehab. WTS's explicitly women-centered mission and hybrid role in the penal system made it a good candidate. I spoke with WTS's deputy director about volunteering in early 2004, explaining my academic interest in learning how the system treats women. She welcomed me and assigned me to help Patricia, director of the Restabilization Program. I performed tasks such as filing and typing notes during staff meetings. WTS's generous staff members were happy to help me with my education by letting me sit in on therapeutic groups and talking with me about their work. After a short time, I asked Patricia if I could do research at WTS for a paper required by my doctoral program, and she said yes. While doing this pilot research, I decided to expand the study beyond my course paper and obtained approval to do so from New York University's institutional review board (IRB). I stopped volunteering at WTS at this point, as required by the IRB, and completed my research in 2005. My time at WTS raised questions that this case study alone could not answer. WTS's narratives about clients and treatment practices did not easily fit with theories of gendered governance or contemporary punishment. I wondered how punishment shaped therapeutic governance and how addiction operated as a governmentality. How would addiction treatment play out in a nonpenal context? How do larger patterns of governance and the penal state shape institutions' efforts to regulate women? To research these questions, I added a comparison site, and the resulting analysis was the basis for my doctoral dissertation.

I learned a great deal about the rehab field while looking for my second case study. I used the Internet to search for addiction treatment programs in the same northeastern state as WTS.[4] To examine my research questions, I had to use a second program that was all-women and residential like WTS, but that did not have contracts with the criminal justice system or accept government funding. Otherwise, the more similar it was to WTS, the better. Finding a facility that met these criteria was not easy. In part this is because most rehab programs are mixed-sex, especially those outside the criminal justice system. In addition, the treatment field is so entangled with the state that private-pay programs are in the minority. State regulations prevent programs from discriminating based on criminal history, so the distinction between penal and not rests in funding and referral networks. Yet many rehabs have complex funding arrangements with multiple public and private sources. In addition, many programs do not describe their funding on their websites, nor is this information compiled by the state. I learned to read the subtext of program websites to identify likely private-pay programs. Because of the racial and class patterns in punishment, I suspected that such programs would treat people of higher socioeconomic status than WTS did, but I did not seek this difference in clientele. Instead, I was interested in how systems of governance and inequality would shape the client population at the two sites, and thus I approached this difference as a finding. Plenty of rather upscale programs do take government grants. One employee of a rehab I called explained to me that the real distinction was whether a program accepted Medicaid, something Lodge staff members also believed. I found that private-pay programs tend to be relatively luxurious (or present themselves as such). Some specialize in treating people in certain professions, adolescents, or women with eating disorders. Wading through their websites, I saw what the Lodge's competition was. Initially, I had hoped to find a long-term program, which would be a better match for WTS, but I found this to be impossible due to the limits of health insurance reimbursements. Only rehab programs in the orbit of the penal state appear to have long treatment times.

Gaining access as a researcher to institutions that serve relatively privileged people is challenging, which may be why there are so few studies of such places. These organizations are likely to be protective of their own brands and their clients' privacy. Thus power differences made it much easier to access WTS than my second site. I pursued research at three programs and was accepted at Gladstone Lodge in 2008. One of the programs rejected me, and the other showed some tentative interest after I had visited a couple of times. It is possible that the Lodge's acceptance signals that it is an unusual private-pay program. There is no way for me to determine this. However, it is similar to other organizations that have women's programs, uses the dominant twelve-step model, and is funded by mainstream insurance. In addition, the Lodge turned out to be the best fit for my research questions because of its gender-sensitive orientation and the modest class status of its clients. I think that Lodge administrators accepted me because they are proud of the program, and they were flattered that I wanted to study it. (This also seemed to be true at WTS.) In describing my research to Lodge staff members, I explained my questions about how treatment was designed for women and the comparison between the Lodge's program and a criminal justice rehab, but I was careful not to signal any interests that might produce defensiveness, such as my interest in the social construction of addiction and inequality. I did the same at WTS. This kind of partial concealment is necessary in most research, both to gain access and to avoid unduly influencing the situation. Yet it often made me uncomfortable, since I valued participants' worldviews and was grateful that they let me into their lives. Of course, I did influence the situation to a degree, and my research subjects often wondered what I thought. Over time I became more open about my questions and discussed some of my emerging conclusions. Navigating my position in the programs, the privilege I had as a highly educated researcher, and others' impression of me required ongoing reflexivity.

RESEARCH PROCESS AND ANALYSIS

I conducted about seven months of fieldwork at each program, visiting each about two times a week. I continued fieldwork less often for another three to four months. I also returned afterward for interviews and to attend a Lodge "alumni" banquet and a WTS graduation ceremony (tellingly, the Lodge does not have a graduation). At both WTS and the Lodge I gathered data mostly through ethnographic observation of therapeutic group sessions, staff meetings, various events, and other parts of everyday life in the programs. My primary sources were group sessions and staff meetings, but I spent a lot of the in-between time tagging along with my research participants or eating meals or hanging out with them. I also analyzed various therapeutic and administrative documents, and I conducted semistructured interviews with a few staff members. To gain a better grasp on the larger structural and discursive systems that impacted these programs, I supplemented these data by analyzing federal data on funding and admissions patterns, recovery literature, government reports, and documents about initiatives related to treatment, and I charted how the organizations fit in the history of rehab. At the Lodge, I interviewed Ruth, director of the women's program and five other key administrators. I conducted more interviews at the Lodge than at WTS, where my discussions with staff members were usually too informal or drawn out over days to be called interviews. WTS's busy schedule, combined with my reluctance to interfere, made it hard for me to find time to spend with staff members. As my research interests developed with my fieldwork at the Lodge, I hoped to do a round of interviews at WTS in 2008, but I found that nearly all the staff members I had met previously were gone (such organizations often have high turnover). In addition, the organization had undergone such substantial changes that current staffers would not have the same experience as those I had met before. However, I did conduct a follow-up interview with Yvonne, who had been promoted to residential director (the position that Marcus had held). I did not formally interview clients at the Lodge or WTS, but I did talk with many of them at length in more informal contexts.

For ethical and methodological reasons, I was more an observer than a participant. This means that I did not speak in groups unless asked because I did not want to shape the direction of the sessions. I occasionally asked questions at staff meetings, but mostly I listened. I also did not want to wield power over clients. Although I never worked with WTS clients as a volunteer, this concern was part of why I left that role. Rehabs are unequal places, where clients are often in great distress and vulnerable to coercion. Consequently, I did not observe individual counseling sessions. This was one of several restrictions that the IRB placed on my research at WTS, because the clients are considered prisoners. At the Lodge I used the same strategy because it enabled clients to have space outside my research as they carried out their lives in a total institution. Not observing individual counseling sessions certainly hindered my view of the treatment process, but it was an acceptable limitation to ensure that the research did not interfere with treatment or harm clients. Instead, I asked staff members and clients about these sessions.

Not only are clients under varying degrees of coercion, but I also collected very sensitive information. Staff members are also vulnerable as employees. Consequently, I took careful measures to maintain confidentiality; explain the project to clients, some of whom were barely literate; and eliminate possible sources of coercion. A major concern was enabling the clients to decide to participate in my research without pressure. I also wanted to conceal their decisions from the staff, although I had no reason to believe staff members cared whether or not clients participated. To do this, I would present my research and distribute consent forms to clients at house meetings and before groups. Clients could hand me the completed forms at any time. I followed a similar consent procedure with staff members. Because WTS clients are prisoners, I took extra steps to make sure that they could consent (or not) privately, including setting up a drop box where they could leave the signed consent forms. If individuals did not consent to participate, I did not write down what they said or did. Because I started at WTS as a volunteer, I was anxious during my process of coming out as a researcher. Changing roles was a long and uneven process given the fast pace of life at WTS and the turnover in the client population. Concerns about confidentiality also led me to conceal the state where I conducted research. While this regional and governmental context is important to a full understanding of WTS and the Lodge, they could be identified by someone with knowledge of the state's treatment field.

I wrote my fieldnotes at the end of each day and transcribed the notes I had taken during meetings. Since I did not take notes in most therapeutic group sessions, I do not have many direct quotations from them. What I put in quotation marks are actual quotations. After writing a detailed narrative of what I had observed, I concluded each day's fieldnotes by stepping back to write analytic memos on what I had observed. These served as the basis for finding patterns, generating further questions, and developing connections between data and theory. From them I added new concepts, patterns, and categories to the list of codes I had generated from existing theory and research on punishment and gendered governance. My fieldwork at WTS created a framework for me to start analyzing my data from the Lodge. After my time at the Lodge, I returned with new ideas and recoded my WTS fieldnotes and documents. I manually coded most of my fieldnotes, interviews, and other documents. In addition, I used the qualitative data analysis program Atlas TI for some notes and transcripts. While in the field, I would check certain things that one person told me with other people. However, my goal was not always to determine who or what was right, but to unearth the interpretive frameworks and narratives that people used. One ongoing difficulty I faced was the dramatic inconsistency within staff narratives about clients, most notably at the Lodge. But what appeared to me as incoherence did not trouble the counselors. In the end, it was the coexistence and interaction of various frameworks that I needed to understand and situate in the larger context where staff members worked. As I became increasingly critical of both programs, I also faced the challenge of making sociologically understandable the ideas and practices that I found problematic. It was easy to just point out a practice and say it was bad. It was also easy to have knee-jerk sympathy for the clients and paint staff members as bad agents of social control, a common trope in studies of such institutions. I needed to take the staff members' perspectives and decisions seriously, although I remained critical of them. To analyze the staff I delved more deeply into the structure and discourses of the rehab field and how they shaped the treatment process. This was an enormously fruitful path. When I began my research with questions about punishment, governance, race, and gender, I did not intend to focus so much on the construction and uses of the term "addiction." It was my attempt to make sense of counselors' practices and organizational dynamics that made this such a central part of my analysis and enabled me to identify the phenomenon of governing through addiction.

POWER AND POSITIONALITY

We can never escape social inequalities when doing research, and they affected both my role as a researcher and my relationships with participants. Yet inequality and insider-outsider dynamics shifted depending on the situation, the individuals involved, and across sites in some unpredictable ways. I was typically more privileged than the staff members and clients at both programs due to my education, middle-class background, and (at WTS) my whiteness. Moreover, as a researcher and neophyte to the rehab world, I was an outsider in other ways. I was very conscious of racial and class differences throughout my fieldwork. In my fieldnotes, I regularly reflected on my positionality and its influence on my interpretations. Yet treating participants with respect and gaining meaningful rapport with them required that I not exoticize them or our differences. I generally managed my outsider status by not concealing my background or past, while also being engaged and easygoing. I tried not to interfere or seem like a know-it-all. In interactions with my research participants, I made sure to show them that I wanted to learn from them by listening and asking questions. For reasons that will become clearer, I avoided any official roles, intervening in conflicts, or giving advice. Lodge clients and staff did occasionally ask my opinion or seek my affirmation in moments of indignation. Not responding in the normal fashion made me a frustrating conversationalist at times.

At WTS, I stood out from the majority of clients and staff in all ways but gender. This social distance could make my goals and social location confusing. People often mistook me for an undergraduate student or someone in training to be a counselor. Such misunderstandings often continued even after I tried to clarify my role. However, WTS had several staff members with advanced degrees who certainly understood my position. My class status and race especially shaped my relationship with WTS clients, whom I got to know less well than Lodge clients. This was also due to the greater time I spent with clients at the Lodge and my ability to stay overnight in the women's unit there. Yet at the same time, WTS women seemed much less perturbed by my presence than Lodge clients were. This was because WTS clients had long experience with surveillance from more powerful people. No amount of easygoingness on my part could change this fact. But many of them were quite eager to talk to me once they understood my role. I think they were happy to have someone who was neither a staff member nor a fellow client to talk with—even about minor things. It was a break from the much higher-stakes surveillance that permeated their everyday life. WTS clients were also quite savvy about the organization's dynamics, and it was quickly obvious to them that I had no power with the staff. Despite large social differences, I blended in better at WTS than at the Lodge. WTS regularly had social work interns and volunteers. People there thus had available roles to put me in. For many, I was one of several young, white, do-gooder women at the facility and not particularly important. At other times, my relative youth (I was in my midtwenties) made me harder for WTS clients to place, and several women asked me if I was also a client. I was never mistaken for a client at the Lodge.

As I described in the introduction, my race and class background were certainly part of the reason why I had greater access at the Lodge than at WTS. It eased my entry into the intimate, familial culture. My social position enabled Faye to speak openly with me about the people she thought were unworthy of her program. Presumed racial identification also led some white clients at both WTS and the Lodge to feel comfortable expressing racist sentiments to me or appealing to our shared whiteness to foster camaraderie against black women. Because of my role as a researcher, I did not challenge these comments, but biting my tongue was not easy for me. Dynamics of difference and privilege help explain why black women at the Lodge were less likely to consent to participate in my research than were white or Latina clients. Although I had more access at the Lodge, I often felt more like an outsider there than I did at WTS. This was for a couple of reasons. Everyone at the Lodge saw me as alien because I have no history of addiction—an identity that tied counselors and clients together and served as the basis for the treatment regime. In addition, the Lodge had no volunteers or interns. The absence of such people is a sign of the higher social status and greater wealth of the program's clients, compared those at WTS. And Lodge counselors were more uncomfortable being studied than were WTS staff members. These factors combined to make me nearly unintelligible at the Lodge. As neither client nor staff member, I really stood out. The Lodge marked this by requiring me to wear a sticker with the word "visitor" each day. Thus, my presence in the cloistered women's unit regularly confused clients and staff members alike. When the head of housekeeping first saw me, she snapped, "Are you part of this fellowship?"

Power dynamics are important in any social research, but they are particularly acute in institutions like the ones I studied. Race and class were not the only divisions in play. As an ethnographer in organizations where some people have power over others, I had to navigate this challenging divide. The power inequities between clients and staff shaped my research practices and the kind of information I could gather. Affiliating myself with one group could come at the expense of my relationships with the other. I felt this dilemma acutely when choosing what to wear. Dressing professionally linked me to the staff, and wearing casual clothes made me more similar to the clients. This was especially true at the Lodge, given its more conservative norms for employees. Clients may have been just as covered up as the staff, but they were always in casual dress. In contrast, some WTS clients dressed nicely for work and because staff encouraged this. Since my research was on the organizations' governmental practices and I depended on staff members' good-will for access, I usually threw my lot in with the counselors. This meant that I spent more time with staff members than with clients, especially at WTS. As for clothing, I tried to look presentable at WTS but not especially formal. At the Lodge, I felt obligated to dress professionally to have access to the staff meetings. This strongly affiliated me with the staff. Once when I stayed overnight and changed into jeans and a sweatshirt for the evening, Alexa and Susan teased me by saying that I had become like them, thus joining the clients' supposedly lower rank.

My apparent alignment with staff clearly made clients suspicious that I would inform on them. What is more, my role as a researcher and my race and class status made clients worry that I would look down on them. But these factors did not always hurt our relationships. After Alexa and Susan's comment, they proceeded to complain to me about staff surveillance and to mock some counselors. It took time, but I eventually earned the trust of clients at both programs—especially those at the Lodge. For example, Lodge clients regularly allowed me to join them on their walks while they were sneaking cigarettes. I heard less from WTS clients about what staff called "deviations," which makes sense since the risks of discovery were so great. Clients' trust was likewise patterned by race, class, and age, but not exclusively. And I made a special effort to push against these seemingly natural affiliations by spending time with older women and those who were not white. I also gained a special rapport with WTS women in the deeply personal therapeutic groups that I visited continuously, such as the parenting class. To circumvent the fear that I would morally judge them, I felt it was important to explain to clients that my research was not about how they had "gone wrong," nor was I interested in unearthing embarrassing parts of their past. In addition, I made it clear that I would not inform on them, although they probably did not all believe me. Because of the power differences between staff and clients, I was careful about what interpretations I revealed to staff. Maintaining this boundary made my own conduct less egalitarian and cooperative. However, clients often returned to the programs and could be identifiable, and staff members' jobs were at stake. I decided that this was the ethical course.

ACKNOWLEDGMENTS

THIS BOOK is the product of many years of work, and I could not have finished it without the help, support, and inspiration of many people. First and foremost, I owe deep thanks to the clients and staff members at Women's Treatment Services and Gladstone Lodge. They generously let me into their lives and answered my questions. Although I am often critical of the programs, I learned much from their staff members and hope that these pages show my respect for the difficult work that we ask them to do. To them, I am forever grateful.

I began this project while I was a doctoral student at New York University (NYU). There I found wonderful mentors who taught me well and laid the foundation for this book. To my brilliant advisor, Lynne Haney: Your intellectual clarity, feminist theoretical rigor, and keen ethnographic eye provided inspiration from the get-go. You believed in me and took my thinking seriously. This sustained me through graduate school and beyond. Thank you for teaching me to be a sociologist. I also owe more than I can say to David Garland: You brought me into the sociological study of punishment and expanded my scholarly horizons. The unflagging encouragement and incisive advice I received from you helped make this book what it is.

I also benefited from the inspiration and advice of many others. As I developed my analysis, Kelly Hannah-Moffat, Dana Britton, Jill McCorkel, and an anonymous reviewer of my manuscript provided invaluable insights and critiques. Jill in particular offered detailed reading, feedback, and enthusiasm for my work that I appreciate deeply. You are an inspiration. I also could not have completed this project if not for the ongoing camaraderie of, thoughtful comments from, and enlivening discussions with Poulami Roychowdhury, Miranda March, Kerwin Kaye, and Teresa Gowan. They are brilliant scholars who continue to shape me. Ruth Horowitz has been there since the beginning, and her guidance during my early stumblings, especially about the self's relation to others, helped me enormously. Rayna Rapp was formative in the conception of this research and helped with the ethnographic process. As a doctoral student, I had conversations with Deirdre Royster, David Greenberg, Eric Klinenberg, Jeff Manza, Steven Lukes, Harvey Molotoch, Lee Clarke, and

Jo Dixon that made this project better. Emily Mann, Alexandra Cox, Reuben Jonathan Miller, Robert Werth, Nicole Lindhal, Armando Lara-Millán, and Colleen Hackett all helped shape my thinking on punishment and contemporary governance. In addition, my path to this study and commitment to feminist sociology owes much to the inspiration and training of Lynn Chancer, my undergraduate advisor. If not for her, this book would not exist.

Since the early stages of my research, I was lucky to have colleagues at my side whose friendship and intellectual support was invaluable. Jill Conte and Alton Phillips excited and pushed me with their astute sociological minds. Our regular beer outings offered solace and fun. I couldn't have done it without you. Sarah Damaske, Sheera Olasky, Ashley Mears, Amy LeClair, Jenna Appelbaum Newman, Dorit Geva, Ailsa Craig, Tey Meadow, and other members of NYU's Gender Workshop offered comments that shaped my analysis in its early days. I also benefited from the advice and friendship of Christine Scott-Hayward, Issa Kohler-Hausmann, Leslie-Ann Bolden, Michael Friedson, Monika Krause, and Sarah Kaufman. Since coming to Bard College, I have been overwhelmed with joy at the friends I have made. Writing a book is a long and hard process. These people sustained me through this process and believed in me when I didn't. For both your friendship and enriching my intellectual life, I thank Dina Ramadan, Maria Cecire, Jennifer Derr, Jon Anjaria, Michelle Murray, Kritika Yegnashankaran, Ulka Anjaria, Peter Klein, Christian Crouch, Sarah Egan, David Madden, and Clement Thery.

My research at Gladstone Lodge was funded by NYU's Mainzer Pre-Doctoral Research Fellowship. It would not have been possible without this support. I also am grateful for the support of members of Bard's Sociology Program, especially Yuval Elmelech, who has made Bard a wonderful place to work. In addition, I thank Josh Aleksanyan and Kyle Gipson, my fabulous students and research assistants at Bard. Students in my courses on punishment, gender, and deviance always get me thinking in productive ways and remind me why this kind of work matters.

Portions of this book appeared previously in "'Getting Gut-Level': Punishment, Gender, and Therapeutic Governance," *Gender & Society* 22, no. 3 (2008): 303–23, ©2008 Sociologists for Women in Society. Other sections appeared in "Roxanne's Dress: Governing Gender and Marginality through Addiction Treatment," *Signs: Journal of Women in Culture and Society* 39, no. 2 (2014), ©2013 the University of Chicago. I am grateful for permission to use this material.

My editor at Rutgers University Press, Peter Mickulas, has been a more enthusiastic backer than I could have hoped for. I am grateful for his patience and care with this book. His efforts helped me finish and improved my work.

My curiosity about the world and scholarly inclinations began with influence of my father, Rick McKim; my mother, Trish Hickling; my late stepfather, Jim Searing; and my late stepmother, Karen Jaehne. Their intellectual fires burn bright; they set me on this path and trained me well. I could not have finished this book without the care work and encouragement of my mother during the writing process. I sequestered myself with her at our family's house in Nova Scotia, and it was the best "postdoctoral fellowship" I could have asked for. The friendship and support of my sister, Charlotte Kent, and my brothers, Alexander and Keith Searing, mean the world to me. The kindness and enthusiasm I received from Ellen Mittenthal, Sara Hickling, and Bill Gazzard helped me keep going, even at the hardest times. I also want to thank my friend Cody Watson. My feminist consciousness and sociological imagination owe much to your sharp mind and rich experience.

I owe the greatest debt to Damon Root, my partner and husband. You proofread my work, offered writing advice, and pushed me intellectually. My thinking is the better for your influence. Throughout the long process that led to this book, I depended on your unconditional support, ongoing sacrifice, and commitment to equality. Your love and your unfailing belief in me and the value of my work are the greatest gifts I have ever received. Moreover, your intellect, kindness, and ethical commitments will always inspire me. Thank you.

Notes

INTRODUCTION: REHAB IS THE NEW BLACK

1. The names of all individuals and organizations have been changed to protect the participants' confidentiality. In addition, I have modified a small number of inconsequential details about the programs because otherwise they could identify the facilities.
2. The handout was copied from Anonymous, *Twenty-Four Hours a Day* (Center City, MN: Hazeldon Foundation, 1975), September 11.
3. In this book, I use the term "drug" to refer to illegal drugs, alcohol, and pharmaceuticals unless further specification is important. I combine these substances because treatment programs, including the two in this study, do not differentiate among substances when defining addiction. Although people may use specific terms like "alcoholism," it was a truism at both programs that "a drug is a drug is a drug."
4. National Institute on Drug Abuse, "Drugs, Brains, and Behavior: The Science of Addiction" (Bethesda, MD: National Institute on Drug Abuse), NIH Pub No. 10–5605, July 2014, accessed November 4, 2016, https://www.drugabuse.gov/publications/drugs-brains-behavior-science-addiction/drug-abuse-addiction.
5. Despite being a penal institution, WTS refers to the program's residents as "clients." Lodge staff members do so, too. I decided to use this term for the women at both WTS and the Lodge because that is how people at both sites talked. For WTS this term is partially misleading, and it rhetorically deemphasizes the facility's role in punishment.
6. This conceptualization draws on Michel Foucault's concept of "governmentality," which refers to forms of power that operate through shaping and guiding conduct rather than overt force. For example, see Michel Foucault, "Governmentality," in *The Foucault Effect: Studies in Governmentality*, ed. Graham Burchell, Colin Gordon, and Peter Miller (Chicago: University of Chicago Press, 1991).
7. Drug policies played a key role in mass incarceration. See: Marc Mauer, "The Causes and Consequences of Prison Growth in the United States," *Punishment and Society* 3, no. 1 (2001); Bruce Western, *Punishment and Inequality in America* (New York: Russell Sage Foundation, 2007).
8. Ryan Teague Beckwith, "Transcript: Read the Full Text of the Second Republican Debate." Time. September 18, 2015, accessed September 30, 2016, http://time.com/4037239/second-republican-debate-transcript-cnn/.
9. As of March 2016, at least fifteen states require some kind of drug testing or screening for recipients of public assistance, and at least seventeen states have proposed such legislation. See National Conference of State Legislatures, "Drug Testing for Welfare Recipients and Public Assistance" (Denver, CO: National Conference of State Legislatures, March 28, 2016), accessed November 1, 2016, http://www.ncsl.org/research/human-services/drug-testing-and-public-assistance.aspx. For an influential model of gender-responsive treatment for women, see Barbara Bloom, Barbara Owen, and Stephanie Covington, "Gender-Responsive Strategies: Research,

Practice, and Guiding Principles for Women Offenders" (Washington: National Institute of Corrections, 2003). Finally, the Robert Wood Johnson Foundation is only one prominent advocate of incorporating treatment into welfare policy. See Dennis McCarty, K. John McConnell, and Laura A. Schmidt, "Policies for the Treatment of Alcohol and Drug Use Disorders: A Research Agenda for 2010–2015 (Highlights)" (Princeton, NJ: Robert Wood Johnson Foundation, October 2009), accessed September 30, 2016, http://www.rwjf.org/content/dam/farm/reports/reports/2009/rwjf46848.

10. Popular and scientific writing has recently framed junk food as more addictive than cocaine. For example, see Robert H. Lustig, "The Most Unhappy of Pleasures: This Is Your Brain on Sugar," *Atlantic*, February 21, 2012, accessed November 4, 2016, http://www.theatlantic.com/health/archive/2012/02/the-most-unhappy-of-pleasures-this-is-your-brain-on-sugar/253341/. Michael Moss's best-selling book *Salt, Sugar, Fat: How the Food Giants Hooked Us* (New York: Random House, 2013) describes processed foods as addictive and suggests that manufacturers intentionally use the ingredients listed in the title to hook consumers into consuming processed food.

11. Micki McGee, *Self-Help, Inc.: Makeover Culture in American Life* (New York: Oxford University Press, 2005); Substance Abuse and Mental Health Services Administration, "Participation in Self-Help Groups for Alcohol and Illicit Drug Use: 2006 and 2007" (Rockville, MD: Substance Abuse and Mental Health Services Administration, December 30, 2008), accessed September 30, 2016, https://www.orange-papers.org/OAS.SAMHSA.GOV—selfHelp.htm; Trysh Travis, *The Language of the Heart: A Cultural History of the Recovery Movement from Alcoholics Anonymous to Oprah Winfrey* (Chapel Hill: University of North Carolina Press, 2009).

12. Nancy Campbell, *Using Women: Gender, Drug Policy, and Social Justice* (New York: Routledge, 2000); Patricia Hill Collins, *Black Feminist Thought: Knowledge, Consciousness, and the Politics of Empowerment*, 2nd ed. (New York: Routledge, 2000); Sharon Hays, *Flat Broke with Children: Women in the Age of Welfare Reform* (New York: Oxford University Press, 2004); Drew Humphries, *Crack Mothers: Pregnancy, Drugs, and the Media* (Columbus: Ohio State University Press, 1999); Dorothy Roberts, *Killing the Black Body: Race, Reproduction, and the Meaning of Liberty* (New York: Vintage, 1998).

13. The first authors to use this term were John S. Goldkamp, Michael D. White, and Jennifer B. Robinson, in "Do Drug Courts Work? Getting Inside the Drug Court Black Box" (*Journal of Drug Issues* 31, no. 1 [2001]), and Jeff Bouffard and Faye Taxman, in "Looking Inside the 'Black Box' of Drug Court Treatment Services Using Direct Observations" (*Journal of Drug Issues* 34, no. 1 [2004]).

14. Anne Fletcher describes how one famous addiction researcher, Alan Marlatt of the University of Washington, was unable to answer a reporter's questions about what was Lindsay Lohan's rehab program would be like (*Inside Rehab: The Surprising Truth about Addiction Treatment—and How to Get Help That Works* [New York: Viking, 2013], 7).

15. Harry G. Levine, "The Discovery of Addiction: Changing Conceptions of Habitual Drunkenness in America," *Journal of Studies on Alcohol* 39, no. 1 (1978); Mariana Valverde, *Diseases of the Will: Alcohol and the Dilemmas of Freedom* (New York: Cambridge University Press, 1998); Darin Weinberg, *Of Others Inside: Insanity, Addiction, and Belonging in America* (Philadelphia: Temple University Press, 2005).

16. Lance Dodes and Zachary Dodes, *The Sober Truth: Debunking the Bad Science Behind 12-Step Programs and the Rehab Industry* (Boston: Beacon, 2014); Fletcher, *Inside Rehab*; McCarty, McConnell, and Schmidt, "Policies for the Treatment of Alcohol and Drug Use Disorders."

17. Peter Conrad and Joseph Schneider, *Deviance and Medicalization: From Badness to Sickness* (Philadelphia: Temple University Press, 1992).

18. See, for example, Andrew Cohen, "How White Users Made Heroin a Public-Health Problem," *Atlantic*, August 12, 2015, accessed November 5, 2016, http://www.theatlantic.com/politics/archive/2015/08/crack-heroin-and-race/401015/; Marc Mauer, "Our Compassion for Drug Users Should Not Be Determined by Race," *Guardian*, January 7, 2016; Ekow Yankah, "When Addiction Has a White Face," *New York Times*, February 9, 2016.

19. Michel Foucault, *Discipline and Punish: The Birth of the Prison*, trans. Alan Sheridan (New York: Vintage, 1977); David Garland, *Punishment and Welfare: A History of Penal Strategies* (Aldershot, UK: Gower, 1985); David Rothman, *The Discovery of the Asylum: Social Order and Disorder in the New Republic, rev. ed.* (New York: Aldine de Gruyter, 2002).

20. David Garland, *The Culture of Control: Crime and Social Order in Contemporary Society* (Chicago: University of Chicago Press, 2001) 53. See also David Garland, *Punishment and Modern Society: A Study in Social Theory* (Chicago: University of Chicago Press, 1990).

21. Garland, *The Culture of Control*, 27.

22. Erving Goffman, *Asylums: Essays on the Social Situation of Mental Patients and Other Inmates* (New York: Anchor, 1961), 4; Foucault, *Discipline and Punish*.

23. Nikolas Rose, *Governing the Soul: The Shaping of the Private Self*, 2nd ed. (New York: Free Association, 1999).

24. Katherine Beckett, *Making Crime Pay: Law and Order in Contemporary American Politics* (New York: Oxford University Press, 1999); Mauer, "The Causes and Consequences of Prison Growth in the United States"; Craig Reinarman and Harold Levine, *Crack in America: Demon Drugs and Social Justice* (Berkeley: University of California Press, 1997).

25. Michelle Alexander, *The New Jim Crow: Mass Incarceration in the Age of Colorblindness* (New York: New Press, 2012); Beckett, *Making Crime Pay*; Garland, *The Culture of Control*; Jill McCorkel, "Criminally Dependent? Gender, Punishment, and the Rhetoric of Welfare Reform," *Social Politics* 11, no. 3 (2004); Loïc Wacquant, "Deadly Symbiosis: When Ghetto and Prison Meet and Merge," in *Mass Imprisonment: Social Causes and Consequences*, ed. David Garland (London: Sage, 2001).

26. Sentencing Project, "Fact Sheet: Trends in U.S. Corrections" (Washington: Sentencing Project, December 2015), accessed September 30, 2016, http://sentencingproject.org/wp-content/uploads/2016/01/Trends-in-US-Corrections.pdf.

27. The rates per 100,000 people were 760 in 2008 and 680 in 2014. See Danielle Kaeble, Lauren Glaze, Anastasios Tsoutis, and Todd Minton, "Correctional Populations in the United States, 2014" (Washington: Bureau of Justice Statistics, January 21, 2016), accessed September 30, 2016, http://www.bjs.gov/content/pub/pdf/cpus14.pdf; Heather C. West and William J. Sabol, "Prison Inmates at Midyear 2008—Statistical Tables" (Washington: Bureau of Justice Statistics, March 2009), accessed September 30, 2016, http://www.bjs.gov/content/pub/pdf/pim08st.pdf, 16.

28. During my research this number was over 5 million. By 2014, 4.7 million were under community supervision. See Kaeble et al., "Correctional Populations in the United States, 2014."

29. Western, *Punishment and Inequality in America*.

30. Ibid.; Jeff Manza and Christopher Uggen, *Locked Out: Felon Disenfranchisement and American Democracy* (New York: Oxford University Press, 2008).

31. Devah Pager, *Marked: Race, Crime, and Finding Work in an Era of Mass Incarceration* (Chicago: University of Chicago Press, 2007).

32. For women born in 2001, black women have a 1 in 18 lifetime chance of incarceration, compared to 1 in 45 for Hispanic women and 1 in 111 for white women. See Sentencing Project, "Fact Sheet: Trends in U.S. Corrections" (Washington:

Sentencing Project, December 2015), accessed Novermber 1, 2016, http://sentenc-ingproject.org/wp-content/uploads/2016/01/Trends-in-US-Corrections.pdf.

33. Lauren E. Glaze, "Correctional Populations in the United States, 2009" (Washing-ton: Bureau of Justice Statistics, December 2010), accessed September 30, 2016, http://bjs.gov/content/pub/pdf/cpus09.pdf.

34. Deborah A. Frank, Marilyn Augustyn, Wanda Grant Knight, Tripler Pell, and Barry Zuckerman, "Growth, Development, and Behavior in Early Childhood Following Prenatal Cocaine Exposure: A Systematic Review," *Journal of the American Medical Association* 285, no. 12 (2001).

35. Humphries, *Crack Mothers.*

36. House Select Committee on Children, Youth, and Families, *Born Hooked; Confront-ing the Impact of Perinatal Substance Abuse* (Washington: Congress, 1989), accessed November 5, 2016, http://files.eric.ed.gov/fulltext/ED314920.pdf, 156. See also Jeanne Flavin, *Our Bodies, Our Crimes: The Policing of Women's Reproduction in America* (New York: New York University Press, 2009); Roberts, *Killing the Black Body.*

37. Quoted in Jeanne Flavin and Lynn M. Paltrow, "Punishing Pregnant Drug-Using Women: Defying Law, Medicine, and Common Sense," *Journal of Addictive Diseases* 29, no. 2 (2010): 232.

38. Laura Gomez, *Misconceiving Mothers: Legislators, Prosecutors, and the Politics of Prenatal Drug Exposure* (Philadelphia: Temple University Press, 1997).

39. Since being pregnant while using is not itself a crime (except since 2014 in Ten-nessee), these women were charged with a variety of offenses. See Lynn M. Paltrow and Jeanne Flavin, "Arrests of and Forced Interventions on Pregnant Women in the United States, 1973–2005: Implications for Women's Legal Status and Public Health," *Journal of Health Politics, Policy and Law* 38, no. 2 (2013).

40. Ira J. Chasnoff, Harvey J. Landress, and Mark E. Barrett, "The Prevalence of Illicit-Drug or Alcohol Use during Pregnancy and Discrepancies in Mandatory Reporting in Pinellas County, Florida," *New England Journal of Medicine* 322, no. 17 (1990).

41. For two prominent examples, see Malcolm Feeley and Jonathan Simon, "The New Penology: Notes on the Emerging Strategy of Corrections and Its Implications," *Criminology* 30, no. 4 (1992); Wacquant, "Deadly Symbiosis."

42. Katherine Beckett and Naomi Murakawa, "Mapping the Shadow Carceral State: Toward an Institutionally Capacious Approach to Punishment," *Theoretical Criminol-ogy* 16, no. 2 (2012).

43. Hays, *Flat Broke with Children.*

44. Loïc Wacquant, *Punishing the Poor: The Neoliberal Government of Social Insecurity* (Dur-ham, NC: Duke University Press, 2009).

45. Jonathan Simon, *Governing through Crime: How the War on Crime Transformed American Democracy and Created a Culture of Fear* (New York: Oxford University Press, 2007).

46. See, for example, Katherine Beckett and Bruce Western, "Governing Social Margin-ality: Welfare, Incarceration, and the Transformation of State Policy," in *Mass Impris-onment: Social Causes and Consequences,* ed. David Garland (London: Sage, 2001); Issa Kohler-Hausmann, "Misdemeanor Justice: Control without Conviction," *American Journal of Sociology* 119, no. 2 (2013); Wacquant, "Deadly Symbiosis."

47. Feeley and Simon (in "The New Penology") and other scholars have noted the rise of risk management in the penal system. Simon (in *Governing through Crime*) expands this to show how risk management techniques are used to manage crime and disorder in other sites of governance.

48. Michelle Phelps argues that rehabilitative services have persisted but they do look different, with less education and more life-skills programs ("Rehabilitation in the Punitive Era: The Gap between Rhetoric and Reality in US Prison Programs," *Law & Society Review* 45, no. 1 [2011]).

49. Kerwin Kaye, "Drug Courts and the Treatment of Addiction: Therapeutic Jurisprudence and Neoliberal Governance," PhD diss., New York University, 2010; Gwen Robinson, "Late-Modern Rehabilitation: The Evolution of a Penal Strategy," *Punishment and Society* 10, no. 4 (2008).

50. Kelly Hannah-Moffat, "Criminogenic Needs and the Transformative Risk Subject: Hybridizations of Risk/Need in Penality," *Punishment and Society* 7, no. 1 (2005); "Assembling Risk and the Restructuring of Penal Control," *British Journal of Criminology* 46 (2006).

51. Jill McCorkel, *Breaking Women: Gender, Race, and the New Politics of Imprisonment* (New York: New York University Press, 2013), 73.

52. Substance Abuse and Mental Health Services Administration, "National Survey of Substance Abuse Treatment Services (NSSATS): 2010: Data on Substance Abuse Treatment Facilities" (Rockville, MD: Substance Abuse and Mental Health Services Administration, September 2011), accessed September 30, 2016, http://wwwdasis.samhsa.gov/10nssats/NSSATS2010Web.pdf; and "Treatment Episode Data Set (TEDS): 2000–2010: National Admissions to Substance Abuse Treatment Services" (Rockville, MD: Substance Abuse and Mental Health Services Administration, June 2012), accessed September 30, 2016, http://wwwdasis.samhsa.gov/dasis2/teds_pubs/2010_teds_rpt_natl.pdf.

53. These percentages do not include facilities that receive payments from Medicaid or Medicare. This analysis is based on data from the Center for Behavioral Health Statistics and Quality of the Substance Abuse and Mental Health Services Administration. See ICPSR, "National Survey of Substance Abuse Treatment Services (N-SSATS)—Concatenated 1997–2011," accessed November 5, 2016, http://www.icpsr.umich.edu/icpsrweb/ICPSR/studies/28544.

54. Substance Abuse and Mental Health Services Administration, "National Expenditures for Mental Health Services and Substance Abuse Treatment, 1986–2009," (Rockville, MD: Substance Abuse and Mental Health Services Administration, 2013), accessed September 30, 2016, https://store.samhsa.gov/shin/content/SMA13-4740/SMA13-4740.pdf.

55. Robert P. Fairbanks, *How It Works: Recovering Citizens in Post-Welfare Philadelphia* (Chicago: University of Chicago Press, 2009); Lynne Haney, *Offending Women: Gender, Punishment, and the Regulation of Desire* (Berkeley: University of California Press, 2010); McCorkel, *Breaking Women;* Reuben Jonathan Miller, "Devolving the Carceral State: Race, Prisoner Reentry, and the Micro-Politics of Urban Poverty Management," *Punishment and Society* 16, no. 3 (2014) Susan Starr Sered and Maureen Norton-Hawk, *Can't Catch a Break: Gender, Jail, Drugs, and the Limits of Personal Responsibility* (Berkeley: University of California Press, 2014).

56. Some states have tried to make this testing universal and mandatory, but these policies have been overturned by courts on constitutional grounds.

57. National Conference of State Legislatures, "Drug Testing for Welfare Recipients and Public Assistance."

58. Teresa Gowan, *Hobos, Hustlers, and Backsliders: Homeless in San Francisco* (Minneapolis: University of Minnesota Press, 2010).

59. Forrest Stuart, "From 'Rabble Management' to 'Recovery Management': Policing Homelessness in Marginal Urban Space," *Urban Studies* 51, no. 9 (2013).

60. Kelly Hannah-Moffat, "Losing Ground: Gendered Knowledges, Parole Risk, and Responsibility," *Social Politics* 11, no. 3 (2004); and "Moral Agent or Actuarial Subject: Risk and Canadian Women's Imprisonment," *Theoretical Criminology* 3, no. 1 (1999).

61. McCorkel, *Breaking Women.*

62. Bloom, Owen, and Covington, "Gender-Responsive Strategies."

63. Rebecca Tiger, *Judging Addicts: Drug Courts and Coercion in the Justice System* (New York: New York University Press, 2012).

64. McCorkel, *Breaking Women*, x. See also Teresa Gowan and Sarah Whetstone, "Making the Criminal Addict: Subjectivity and Social Control in a Strong-Arm Rehab," *Punishment and Society* 14, no. 1 (2012); Haney, *Offending Women*; Kerwin Kaye, "Rehabilitating the 'Drugs Lifestyle': Criminal Justice, Social Control, and the Cultivation of Agency," *Ethnography* 14, no. 2 (2013).

65. William L. White, *Slaying the Dragon: The History of Addiction Treatment and Recovery in America* (Bloomington, IL: Chestnut Health Systems, 1998).

66. John Steadman Rice, *A Disease of One's Own: Psychotherapy, Addiction, and the Emergence of Co-Dependency* (New Brunswick, NJ: Transaction, 1996); Travis, *The Language of the Heart*. For the concept of "moral entrepreneurs," see Howard Becker, *Outsiders: Studies in the Sociology of Deviance* (New York: Free Press, 1963).

67. Nikolas Rose, *Governing the Soul, and Powers of Freedom: Reframing Political Thought* (Cambridge: Cambridge University Press, 1999).

68. I thank Jill McCorkel for the phrase "suspended citizenship."

69. Kai Erikson, *Wayward Puritans: A Study in the Sociology of Deviance*, rev. ed. (Boston: Pearson/Allyn and Bacon, 2005); Harold Garfinkel, "Conditions of Successful Degradation Ceremonies," *American Journal of Sociology* 61, no. 5 (1956); Garland, *Punishment and Modern Society*.

70. Wacquant, "Deadly Symbiosis," 103.

71. Julia Adams and Tasleem Padamsee, "Signs and Regimes: Rereading Feminist Work on Welfare States," *Social Politics* 8, no. 1 (2001).

72. Julia S. O'Connor, Ann Shola Orloff, and Sheila Shaver, *States, Markets, Families: Gender, Liberalism and Social Policy in Australia, Canada, Great Britain and the United States* (New York: Cambridge University Press, 1999).

73. Nancy Fraser and Linda Gordon, "A Geneaology of Dependency: Tracing a Keyword of the U.S. Welfare State," in *Justice Interruptus*, ed. Nancy Fraser (New York: Routledge, 1997).

74. Nancy Campbell and Elizabeth Ettorre, *Gendering Addiction: The Politics of Drug Treatment in a Neurochemical World* (New York: Palgrave Macmillan, 2011).

75. Jennifer Reich, *Fixing Families: Parents, Power, and the Child Welfare System* (New York: Routledge, 2005); Dorothy Roberts, *Shattered Bonds: The Color of Child Welfare* (New York: Basic Civitas Books, 2002).

76. Faye S. Taxman and Jeffrey Bouffard, "Treatment Inside the Drug Court: The Who, What, Where, and How of Treatment Services," *Substance Use and Misuse* 37, nos. 12–13 (2002): 1666.

77. Sanford Schram, "In the Clinic: The Medicalization of Welfare," *Social Text* 18, no. 1 (2000): 82.

78. Travis, *The Language of the Heart*.

79. Leslie Irvine, *Codependent Forevermore: The Invention of Self in a Twelve Step Group* (Chicago: University of Chicago Press, 1999).

80. Miranda March, "Rubrics of Rehabilitation: Gendered Narratives of Selfhood in Court Mandated Treatment Facilities" (PhD diss., New York University, 2009); Jessica J. B. Wyse, "Rehabilitating Criminal Selves: Gendered Strategies in Community Corrections," *Gender and Society* 27, no. 2 (2013).

81. Gladstone Lodge also runs a program for men, but they are housed separately and treated by different counseling staff.

82. This means I often cannot recount the exact words of the participants. However, any statement in quotation marks is an actual quotation.

CHAPTER I INTAKE: PATHWAYS TO TREATMENT

1. Under the 1997 federal Adoption and Safe Families Act, states must terminate parental custody if a child has been in foster care for fifteen of the previous twenty-two months. This law sought to increase the placement of foster children, but since the median state sentence for nonviolent drug crimes is thirty-six months, it has destroyed the families of many incarcerated parents (mostly women). See Lynn Lu and Patricia Allard, "National Study Faults Federal 'Adoption & Safe Families Act' for Consigning Children to Permanent Separation from Parents" (New York: Brennan Center for Justice, September 7 2006), accessed October 1, 2016, http://www.brennancenter.org/press-release/national-study-faults-federal-adoption-safe-families-act-consigning-children-permanent.

2. Lynne Haney, *Offending Women: Gender, Punishment, and the Regulation of Desire* (Berkeley: University of California Press, 2010); Candace Kruttschnitt and Rose-mary Gartner, *Marking Time in the Golden State: Women's Imprisonment in California* (Cambridge: Cambridge University Press, 2005); Jill McCorkel, *Breaking Women: Gender, Race, and the New Politics of Imprisonment* (New York: New York University Press, 2013).

3. Nancy Campbell and Elizabeth Ettorre, *Gendering Addiction: The Politics of Drug Treatment in a Neurochemical World* (New York: Palgrave Macmillan, 2011); William L. White, *Slaying the Dragon: The History of Addiction Treatment and Recovery in America* (Bloomington, IL: Chestnut Health Systems, 1998).

4. White, *Slaying the Dragon.*

5. Harry G. Levine, "The Discovery of Addiction: Changing Conceptions of Habitual Drunkenness in America," *Journal of Studies on Alcohol* 39, no. 1 (1978): 146. Frequent substance use was first formulated as a disease around 1784 by Benjamin Rush, a signer of the Declaration of Independence, founding father of psychiatry, and early prison reformer. Rush termed the "habitual use of ardent spirits" "an odious disease" and held that chronic drunkenness was characterized by a "loss of willpower" brought on by hard liquor (White, *Slaying the Dragon*, xiii).

6. Levine, "The Discovery of Addiction"; David Rothman, *The Discovery of the Asylum: Social Order and Disorder in the New Republic, rev. ed.* (New York: Aldine de Gruyter, 2002).

7. White, *Slaying the Dragon.*

8. In 1874, the Albany, New York, penitentiary claimed that "more than 6,000 women had been confined there, 'nearly all inebriates'" (ibid., 43).

9. Joseph R. Gusfield, *Symbolic Crusade: Status Politics and the American Temperance Movement, 2nd ed.* (Urbana: University of Illinois Press, 1986).

10. David Musto, *The American Disease: Origins of Narcotics Control*, 3rd ed. (New York: Oxford University Press, 1999); White, *Slaying the Dragon.*

11. Darin Weinberg, *Of Others Inside: Insanity, Addiction, and Belonging in America* (Philadelphia: Temple University Press, 2005). For information on the asylums' population, see White, *Slaying the Dragon.*

12. Mariana Valverde, *Diseases of the Will: Alcohol and the Dilemmas of Freedom* (New York: Cambridge University Press, 1998).

13. Rothman, *Discovery of the Asylum, 133 and 206.*

14. White, *Slaying the Dragon.*

15. Not only did the asylums close, but so did scientific journals and professional associations dedicated to studying inebriety.

16. Valverde, *Diseases of the Will.*

17. White, *Slaying the Dragon*, 67.

18. On the shift to seeing opiate addicts as men, see David T. Courtwright, *Dark Para-dise: A History of Opiate Addiction in America*, enlarged ed. (Cambridge, MA: Harvard University Press, 2001). Yet those men remained gender deviant. See Mara L. Keire, "Dope Fiends and Degenerates: The Gendering of Addiction in the Early Twentieth Century," *Journal of Social History* 31, no. 4 (1998).

19. White, *Slaying the Dragon*.

20. Campbell and Ettorre, *Gendering Addiction*.

21. Trysh Travis, *The Language of the Heart: A Cultural History of the Recovery Movement from Alcoholics Anonymous to Oprah Winfrey* (Chapel Hill: University of North Caro-lina Press, 2009).

22. Nancy Campbell, *Discovering Addiction: The Science and Politics of Substance Abuse Research* (Ann Arbor: University of Michigan Press, 2007); Valverde, *Diseases of the Will*.

23. Campbell and Ettorre, *Gendering Addiction*; Constance Weisner and Robin Room, "Financing and Ideology in Alcohol Treatment," *Social Problems* 32, no. 2 (1984); White, *Slaying the Dragon*.

24. Quoted in Carolyn Wiener, *The Politics of Alcoholism: Building an Arena around a Social Problem* (New Brunswick, NJ: Transaction, 1981), 3.

25. Lance Dodes and Zachary Dodes, *The Sober Truth: Debunking the Bad Science Behind 12-Step Programs and the Rehab Industry* (Boston: Beacon, 2014); Travis, *The Language of the Heart;* White, *Slaying the Dragon.*

26. The Department of Substance Abuse Services (DSAS) license is required for the program to be eligible for insurance coverage. Furthermore, the Lodge participates in a voluntary private certification program for rehabilitation facilities. Along with DSAS, this certification agency performs regular inspections and audits.

27. Substance Abuse and Mental Health Services Administration, "Treatment Episode Data Set (TEDS): 2004–2014: National Admissions to Substance Abuse Treatment Services" (Rockville, MD: Substance Abuse and Mental Health Services Admin-istration, 2016), accessed November 1, 2016, http://www.samhsa.gov/data/sites/default/files/2014_Treatment_Episode_Data_Set_National_Admissions_9_19_16.pdf, 9.

28. Quoted in Travis, *The Language of the Heart, 44.*

29. James A. Walker, "Union Members in 2007: A Visual Essay," *Monthly Labor Review,* October 2008, 28–39, accessed October 1, 2016, http://www.bls.gov/opub/mlr/2008/10/art3full.pdf.

30. These racial/ethnic percentages are based on a combination of clients' self-identification and my own guesses. I did not conduct surveys with the clients that asked them things like their ethnic or racial identification, and I could not get self-reports from all clients while I observed everyday life. Making such evaluations based on visual cues or accents is inherently problematic, and thus these numbers must be regarded as approximate estimates.

31. Marie Gottschalk, *The Shadow Welfare State: Labor, Business, and the Politics of Health-Care in the United States* (Ithaca, NY: Cornell University Press, 2000).

32. Campbell and Ettorre, *Gendering Addiction*.

33. This was especially true of the unions with relatively more money. Vincent noted that people affiliated with the poorer unions, like the Service Employees Inter-national Union, had shorter stays. This disadvantages women, since they are more likely than men to be members of poorer unions.

34. Faye S. Taxman, Matthew L. Perdoni, and Lana D. Harrison, "Drug Treatment Ser-vices for Adult Offenders: The State of the State," *Journal of Substance Abuse Treatment* 32, no. 3 (2007).

35. For data on the funding sources for treatment, see Substance Abuse and Mental Health Services Administration, "National Expenditures for Mental Health Services

and Substance Abuse Treatment, 1986–2009," (Rockville, MD: Substance Abuse and Mental Health Services Administration, 2013), accessed September 30, 2016, https://store.samhsa.gov/shin/content/SMA13-4740/SMA13-4740.pdf.

36. While I conducted fieldwork at WTS, I knew of only two women who were truly voluntary, with neither a criminal justice mandate nor CPS stipulations. WTS had a couple of slots for such women, called "community members."

37. Jennifer Reich, *Fixing Families: Parents, Power, and the Child Welfare System* (New York: Routledge, 2005), 82.

38. Ibid.

39. Dorothy Roberts, *Shattered Bonds: The Color of Child Welfare* (New York: Basic Civitas Books, 2002).

40. The percentages are from WTS's data at the time of my research. According to public data for the program in 2012, several years after my research, the WTS population is about 60 percent African American, 20 percent non-Hispanic white, and 20 percent Hispanic or Latina.

41. Susan Starr Sered and Maureen Norton-Hawk, *Can't Catch a Break: Gender, Jail, Drugs, and the Limits of Personal Responsibility* (Berkeley: University of California Press, 2014).

42. National data also suggest that people referred to a program by the criminal justice system tend to be more privileged than those who reach the program from other pathways: they are more likely to be employed and less likely to be black. However, these data include people mandated through DWI or driving under the influence (DUI) programs, which are likely to deal with people from a wide range of socioeconomic backgrounds. This may also indicate that relatively privileged people are more likely to get rehabilitative sanctions, as Rebecca Tiger suggests (*Judging Addicts: Drug Courts and Coercion in the Justice System* [New York: New York University Press, 2012]). See also Substance Abuse and Mental Health Services Administration, "The TEDs Report: Substance Abuse Treatment Admissions Referred by the Criminal Justice System" (Rockville, MD: Substance Abuse and Mental Health Services Administration, 2009).

43. Teresa Gowan and Sarah Whetstone, "Making the Criminal Addict: Subjectivity and Social Control in a Strong-Arm Rehab," *Punishment and Society* 14, no. 1 (2012); Kerwin Kaye, "Drug Courts and the Treatment of Addiction: Therapeutic Jurisprudence and Neoliberal Governance" (PhD diss., New York University, 2010); McCorkel, *Breaking Women.*

44. The most influential model of gender-specific treatment is described in Barbara Bloom, Barbara Owen, and Stephanie Covington, "Gender-Responsive Strategies: Research, Practice, and Guiding Principles for Women Offenders" (Washington: National Institute of Corrections, 2003). For a history of women's efforts to reform the rehab system, see Campbell and Ettorre, *Gendering Addiction.*

45. Thomas M. Brady and Olivia S. Ashley, "Women in Substance Abuse Treatment: Results from the Alcohol and Drug Services Study (ADSS)" (Rockville, MD: Substance Abuse and Mental Health Service Administration, 2005).

46. Campbell and Ettorre, *Gendering Addiction;* Christine E. Grella, "From Generic to Gender-Responsive Treatment: Changes in Social Policies, Treatment Services, and Outcomes of Women in Substance Abuse Treatment," *Journal of Psychoactive Drugs* 40, supplement 5 (2008).

47. Rachel Porter, Sophia Lee, and Mary Lutz, "Balancing Treatment and Punishment: Alternatives to Incarceration in New York City" (New York: Vera Institute for Justice, 2002).

48. Lynne Haney, "Gender, Welfare, and States of Punishment," *Social Politics* 11, no. 3 (2004); and *Offending Women.*

49. Erving Goffman, *Asylums: Essays on the Social Situation of Mental Patients and Other Inmates* (New York: Anchor, 1961) 12.

CHAPTER 2 WOMEN'S TREATMENT SERVICES:
ADDICTED TO PUNISHMENT

1. Borrowing from Everett C. Hughes's work, Howard Becker has argued that deviant labels can easily become master statuses (*Outsiders: Studies in the Sociology of Deviance* [New York: Free Press, 1963]).
2. While WTS dealt with mostly illegal drug users, the staff considered addiction to encompass all substances, including alcohol. This was true at Gladstone Lodge, too. Accordingly, I use the terms "addict" and "addiction" generically rather than distinguishing between people who use alcohol and those who use other drugs. Moreover, I make no claim about whether these people are really addicts or not. Instead, I use the terms to refer to how the programs defined these individuals.
3. Katherine Beckett and Bruce Western, "Governing Social Marginality: Welfare, Incarceration, and the Transformation of State Policy," in *Mass Imprisonment: Social Causes and Consequences*, ed. David Garland (London: Sage, 2001); Loïc Wacquant, "Deadly Symbiosis: When Ghetto and Prison Meet and Merge," in *Mass Imprisonment*; Bruce Western, *Punishment and Inequality in America* (New York: Russell Sage Foundation, 2007).
4. Jonathan Simon, *Poor Discipline: Parole and the Social Control of the Underclass, 1890–1990* (Chicago: University of Chicago Press, 1993). For an excellent summary of this Marxist tradition, see David Garland, *Punishment and Modern Society: A Study in Social Theory* (Chicago: University of Chicago Press, 1990).
5. Dana M. Britton, *At Work in the Iron Cage: The Prison as a Gendered Organization* (New York: New York University Press, 2003).
6. Ruth M. Alexander, *The "Girl Problem": Female Sexual Delinquency in New York 1900–1930* (Ithaca, NY: Cornell University Press, 1995); Jeanne Flavin, "Of Punishment and Parenthood: Family-Based Social Control and the Sentencing of Black Drug Offenders," *Gender and Society* 15, no. 4 (2001); Nicole Hahn Rafter, *Partial Justice: Women, Prisons, and Social Control* (New Brunswick, NJ: Transaction, 1995).
7. For example, see Michelle Alexander, *The New Jim Crow: Mass Incarceration in the Age of Colorblindness* (New York: New Press, 2012); Malcolm Feeley and Jonathan Simon, "The New Penology: Notes on the Emerging Strategy of Corrections and Its Implications," *Criminology* 30, no. 4 (1992): 449–70; David Garland, *The Culture of Control: Crime and Social Order in Contemporary Society* (Chicago: University of Chicago Press, 2001); Loïc Wacquant, *Punishing the Poor: The Neoliberal Government of Social Insecurity* (Durham, NC: Duke University Press, 2009).
8. While women's prisons remain gendered institutions, recent studies suggest that the penal paternalism is on the wane. See Candace Kruttschnitt and Rosemary Gartner, *Marking Time in the Golden State: Women's Imprisonment in California* (Cambridge: Cambridge University Press, 2005); Jill McCorkel, *Breaking Women: Gender, Race, and the New Politics of Imprisonment* (New York: New York University Press, 2013).
9. Synanon later turned itself into what it called a church and ran into legal trouble for a host of violent and financial crimes.
10. George DeLeon, *The Therapeutic Community: Theory, Model, and Method* (New York: Springer, 2000).
11. McCorkel, *Breaking Women*.
12. New York State Department of Corrections and Community Supervision, "About DOCCS," accessed October 2, 2016, http://www.doccs.ny.gov/.
13. Teresa Gowan and Sarah Whetstone, "Making the Criminal Addict: Subjectivity and Social Control in a Strong-Arm Rehab," *Punishment and Society* 14, no. 1 (2012);

Kerwin Kaye, "Drug Courts and the Treatment of Addiction: Therapeutic Juris-prudence and Neoliberal Governance" (PhD diss., New York University, 2010); McCorkel, *Breaking Women.* In a study of a woman's prison, Lynne Haney did not find that it used the term "habilitation," but the program called itself a TC and oper-ated with similar ideas about addiction (*Offending Women: Gender, Punishment, and the Regulation of Desire* [Berkeley: University of California Press, 2010]).

14. Mariana Valverde, *Diseases of the Will: Alcohol and the Dilemmas of Freedom* (New York: Cambridge University Press, 1998). For an excellent account of how addiction treatment has been woven into the management of the poor, see Darin Weinberg, *Of Others Inside: Insanity, Addiction, and Belonging in America* (Philadelphia: Temple University Press, 2005).

15. Gowan and Whetstone, "Making the Criminal Addict," 69.

16. Kerwin Kaye, "Rehabilitating the 'Drugs Lifestyle': Criminal Justice, Social Control, and the Cultivation of Agency," *Ethnography* 14, no. 2 (2013): 210. On the history of TCs, see Kaye, "Drug Courts and the Treatment of Addiction."

17. Yvonne's comments are supported by studies such as Barbara Bloom, Barbara Owen, and Stephanie Covington, "Gender-Responsive Strategies: Research, Prac-tice, and Guiding Principles for Women Offenders" (Washington: National Institute of Corrections, 2003). For critiques of twelve-step programs for women, see Trysh Travis, *The Language of the Heart: A Cultural History of the Recovery Movement from Alcoholics Anonymous to Oprah Winfrey* (Chapel Hill: University of North Carolina Press, 2009).

18. The two most famous examples are Melody Beattie, *Codependent No More: How to Stop Controlling Others and Start Caring for Yourself* (New York: Harper/Hazelden, 1987), and Robin Norwood, *Women Who Love Too Much: When You Keep Wishing and Hoping He'll Change* (New York: Simon and Schuster, 1986).

19. Leslie Irvine, *Codependent Forevermore: The Invention of Self in a Twelve Step Group* (Chicago: University of Chicago Press, 1999); John Steadman Rice, *A Disease of One's Own: Psychotherapy, Addiction, and the Emergence of Co-Dependency* (New Bruns-wick, NJ: Transaction, 1996); Travis, *The Language of the Heart.*

20. Arlie Hochschild, *The Commercialization of Intimate Life: Notes from Home and Work* (Berkeley: University of California Press, 2003).

21. Caroline Wolf Harlow found that 57.2 percent of women in state prison reported prior abuse, and 36.7 percent of women reported abuse occurring before the age of eighteen ("Prior Abuse Reported by Inmates and Probationers," [Washington: Bureau of Justice Statistics, April 1999], accessed October 2, 2016, https://www.prearesourcecenter.org/sites/default/files/library/priorabusereportedbyinmate-sandprobationers.pdf). These rates are much higher than those reported by male inmates. Another study found that 70 percent of incarcerated women had expe-rienced an assault that would qualify as rape in most states, and about half had experienced childhood sexual abuse, often from male family members. See Cathy McDaniels-Wilson and Joanne Belknap, "The Extensive Sexual Violation and Sexual Abuse Histories of Incarcerated Women," *Violence Against Women* 14, no. 10 (2008).

22. Bureau of Justice Assistance, "Residential Substance Abuse Treatment for State Pris-oners (RSAT) Program," (Washington: Bureau of Justice Assistance, April 2005), accessed October 2, 2016, https://www.ncjrs.gov/pdffiles1/bja/206269.pdf.

23. Margaret told me this; I didn't hear it myself.

24. The others were: no fighting, no stealing, and no weapons. At intake, clients and their counselor sign a sheet that lists the rules and states that clients are required to abide by them.

25. Erving Goffman, *Asylums: Essays on the Social Situation of Mental Patients and Other Inmates* (New York: Anchor Books, 1961).

26. Britton, *At Work in the Iron Cage.*
27. Nancy Fraser and Linda Gordon, "A Genealogy of Dependency: Tracing a Keyword of the U.S. Welfare State," in *Justice Interruptus*, ed. Nancy Fraser (New York: Routledge, 1997), 137.
28. Devah Pager, *Marked: Race, Crime, and Finding Work in an Era of Mass Incarceration* (Chicago: University of Chicago Press, 2007).
29. Poulami Roychowdhury found that women's organizations are especially likely to turn to therapeutic strategies when they have limited capacity to address structural issues ("Desire, Rights, Entitlements: Organizational Strategies in the War on Violence," *Signs* 41, no. 4 [2016]).
30. Michel Foucault, *Discipline and Punish: The Birth of the Prison*, trans. Alan Sheridan (New York: Vintage, 1977).
31. Barbara Cruikshank, *The Will to Empower: Democratic Citizens and Other Subjects* (Ithaca, NY: Cornell University Press, 1999); Nikolas Rose, *Powers of Freedom. Reframing Political Thought* (Cambridge: Cambridge University Press, 1999).
32. Kai Erikson famously made this argument (inspired by Émile Durkheim) in *Wayward Puritans: A Study in the Sociology of Deviance*, rev. ed. (Boston: Pearson/Allyn and Bacon, 2005). For a thorough comparison of these different sociological theories of punishment, see Garland, *Punishment and Modern Society.*
33. Harold Garfinkel, "Conditions of Successful Degradation Ceremonies," *American Journal of Sociology* 61, no. 5 (1956).
34. Goffman, *Asylums, 21.*
35. This is quite common throughout the treatment industry. However, I don't know about Yvonne's or Ayana's history.
36. Patricia Williams, *The Alchemy of Race and Rights* (Cambridge, MA: Harvard University Press, 1991), 219.
37. McCorkel, *Breaking Women, 107.*
38. Haney, *Offending Women*; Kruttschnitt and Gartner, *Marking Time in the Golden State*; Candace Kruttschnitt, Rosemary Gartner, and Amy Miller, "Doing Her Own Time? Women's Responses to Prison in the Context of the Old and the New Penology," *Criminology* 38, no. 3 (2000).
39. Haney, *Offending Women*; Kelly Hannah-Moffat, "Feminine Fortresses: Women-Centered Prisons?," *Prison Journal* 75, no. 2 (1995); and "Prisons That Empower: Neo-Liberal Governance in Canadian Women's Prisons," *British Journal of Criminology* 40 (2000).
40. Colleen Hackett, "Transformative Visions: Governing through Alternative Practices and Therapeutic Interventions at a Women's Reentry Center," *Feminist Criminology* 8, no. 3 (2013): 238.
41. McCorkel, *Breaking Women.*

CHAPTER 3 WOMEN'S TREATMENT SERVICES:
            HABILITATING BROKEN WOMEN

1. These desires were mentioned in a majority of the cases that staff members discussed, but I do not have data that would give a numerical percentage.
2. Michel Foucault and those influenced by him often call these "technologies of the self." These technologies serve to align people with the aims of governing authority by enlisting individuals to shape their own subjectivity. See, for example, Michel Foucault, *The History of Sexuality*, Vol. 3: *The Care of the Self*, trans. Robert Hurley (New York: Vintage, 1986); Nikolas Rose, *Governing the Soul: The Shaping of the Private Self*, 2nd ed. (New York: Free Association, 1999).
3. These are characteristic traits of discipline described in Michel Foucault, *Discipline and Punish: The Birth of the Prison*, trans. Alan Sheridan (New York: Vintage, 1977);

Jill McCorkel, "Embodied Surveillance and the Gendering of Punishment," *Journal of Contemporary Ethnography* 32, no. 1 (2003).
4. Rose, *Governing the Soul*.
5. Mariana Valverde, *Diseases of the Will: Alcohol and the Dilemmas of Freedom* (New York: Cambridge University Press, 1998), 30. See also John Steadman Rice, *A Disease of One's Own: Psychotherapy, Addiction, and the Emergence of Co-Dependency* (New Brunswick, NJ: Transaction, 1996).
6. Leslie Irvine, *Codependent Forevermore: The Invention of Self in a Twelve Step Group* (Chicago: University of Chicago Press, 1999), 7.
7. Robin Norwood, *Women Who Love Too Much: When You Keep Wishing and Hoping He'll Change* (New York: Simon and Schuster, 1986).
8. Jessica J. B. Wyse, "Rehabilitating Criminal Selves: Gendered Strategies in Community Corrections," *Gender and Society* 27, no. 2 (2013).
9. It is likely that this placed considerable pressure on women to have abortions.
10. Sharon Hays, *The Cultural Contradictions of Motherhood* (New Haven, CT: Yale University Press, 1998).
11. The first step in the original twelve-step program of Alcoholics Anonymous reads: "We admitted we were powerless over alcohol—that our lives had become unmanageable" (Alcoholics Anonymous World Services, "The Twelve Steps of Alcoholics Anonymous," revised August 2016, accessed October 2, 2016, http://www.aa.org/assets/en_US/smf-121_en.pdf).
12. Nancy Fraser and Linda Gordon, "A Genealogy of Dependency: Tracing a Keyword of the U.S. Welfare State," in *Justice Interruptus*, ed. Nancy Fraser (New York: Routledge, 1997).
13. For example, see Sara Goodkind, "'You Can Be Anything You Want, but You Have to Believe It': Commercialized Feminism in Gender Specific Programs for Girls," *Signs* 34, no. 2 (2009); Colleen Hackett, "Transformative Visions: Governing through Alternative Practices and Therapeutic Interventions at a Women's Reentry Center," *Feminist Criminology* 8, no. 3 (2013); Lynne Haney, *Offending Women: Gender, Punishment, and the Regulation of Desire* (Berkeley: University of California Press, 2010); Kelly Hannah-Moffat, "Prisons That Empower: Neo-Liberal Governance in Canadian Women's Prisons," *British Journal of Criminology* 40 (2000); Miranda March, "Rubrics of Rehabilitation: Gendered Narratives of Selfhood in Court Mandated Treatment Facilities" (PhD diss., New York University, 2009); Jill McCorkel, "Criminally Dependent? Gender, Punishment, and the Rhetoric of Welfare Reform," *Social Politics* 11, no. 3 (2004); Shoshana Pollack, "'I'm Just Not Good in Relationships': Victimization Discourses and the Gender Regulation of Criminalized Women," *Feminist Criminology* 2 (2007); Wyse, "Rehabilitating Criminal Selves."
14. Arlie Hochschild, *The Commercialization of Intimate Life: Notes from Home and Work* (Berkeley: University of California Press, 2003), 13. Hochschild does not characterize the autonomy-oriented modern self-help books as about codependency, but this framework is the theme that links them.
15. Jennifer Reich, *Fixing Families: Parents, Power, and the Child Welfare System* (New York: Routledge, 2005).
16. Patricia Hill Collins, *Black Feminist Thought: Knowledge, Consciousness, and the Politics of Empowerment*, 2nd ed. (New York: Routledge, 2000); Beth E. Richie, *Arrested Justice: Black Women, Violence, and America's Prison Nation* (New York: New York University Press, 2012); Dorothy Roberts, "Punishing Drug Addicts Who Have Babies: Women of Color, Equality, and the Right of Privacy," *Harvard Law Review* 104, no.7 (1990); and "Racism and Patriarchy in the Meaning of Motherhood," *American University Journal of Gender and Law* 1, no.1 (1993).
17. Collins, *Black Feminist Thought*.

18. Kathryn Edin and Maria Kefalas, *Promises I Can Keep: Why Poor Women Put Mother-hood before Marriage* (Berkeley: University of California Press, 2005); Sandra Enos, *Mothering from the Inside: Parenting in a Women's Prison* (Albany: State University of New York Press, 2001); Kathleen J. Ferraro and Angela M. Moe, "Mothering, Crime, and Incarceration," *Journal of Contemporary Ethnography* 32, no. 1 (2003).

19. Erving Goffman, *The Presentation of Self in Everyday Life* (New York: Anchor, 1959); Candace West and Don Zimmerman, "Doing Gender," *Gender and Society* 1, no. 2 (1987).

20. Pierre Bourdieu, *Outline of a Theory of Practice*, translated by Richard Nice (Cambridge: Cambridge University Press, 1977).

21. Goodkind, "'You Can Be Anything You Want.'"

22. Gresham Sykes, *The Society of Captives: A Study of a Maximum Security Prison* (Princeton, NJ: Princeton University Press, 2007), 63.

23. Lisa Delpit, "The Silenced Dialogue: Power and Pedagogy in Educating Other People's Children," *Harvard Educational Review* 58, no. 3, 1988.

24. Mary Odem, *Delinquent Daughters: Protecting and Policing Adolescent Female Sexual-ity in the United States, 1885–1920* (Chapel Hill: University of North Carolina Press, 1995); Nicole Hahn Rafter, *Partial Justice: Women, Prisons, and Social Control* (New Brunswick, NJ: Transaction, 1995).

25. Kevin K. Gaines, *Uplifting the Race: Black Leadership, Politics, and Culture in the Twentieth Century* (Chapel Hill: University of North Carolina Press, 1996); Geoff Ward, *The Black Child-Savers: Racial Democracy and American Juvenile Justice* (Chicago: University of Chicago Press, 2012).

26. Ward, *The Black Child-Savers.*

27. Gaines, *Uplifting the Race.*

28. Ruth M. Alexander, *The "Girl Problem": Female Sexual Delinquency in New York 1900–1930* (Ithaca, NY: Cornell University Press, 1995); Dana M. Britton, *At Work in the Iron Cage: The Prison as a Gendered Organization* (New York: New York University Press, 2003); Meda Chesney-Lind, "Girls' Crime and Woman's Place: Toward a Feminist Model of Female Delinquency," *Crime and Delinquency* 35, no. 1 (1989); Odem, *Delinquent Daughters*; Rafter, *Partial Justice*; Dorothy Roberts, "Motherhood and Crime," *Social Text* 42 (Spring 1995).

29. See, for example, Tammy L. Anderson, *Neither Villain nor Victim: Empowerment and Agency among Women Substance Abusers* (New Brunswick, NJ: Rutgers University Press, 2008); Nancy Campbell, *Using Women: Gender, Drug Policy, and Social Justice* (New York: Routledge, 2000); Nancy Campbell and Elizabeth Ettorre, *Gendering Addiction: The Politics of Drug Treatment in a Neurochemical World* (New York: Palgrave Macmillan, 2011); Drew Humphries, *Crack Mothers: Pregnancy, Drugs, and the Media* (Columbus: Ohio State University Press, 1999).

30. Patrick Biernacki, *Pathways from Heroin Addiction: Recovery without Treatment* (Philadelphia: Temple University Press, 1986). See also William Cloud and Robert Granfield, and "Conceptualizing Recovery Capital: Expansion of a Theoretical Construct," *Substance Use and Misuse* 43, nos. 12–13 (2008); and "Natural Recovery from Substance Dependency," *Journal of Social Work Practice in the Addictions* 1, no. 1 (2001).

31. Barbara Cruikshank, *The Will to Empower: Democratic Citizens and Other Subjects* (Ithaca, NY: Cornell University Press, 1999), 88.

32. Fraser and Gordon, "A Genealogy of Dependency"; Gwendolyn Mink, "The Lady and the Tramp: Gender, Race, and the Origins of the American Welfare State," in *Women, the State, and Welfare*, ed. Linda Gordon (Madison: University of Wisconsin Press, 1990).

33. For example, see Joanne Belknap, *The Invisible Woman: Gender, Crime, and Justice*, 3rd ed. (Belmont, CA: Wadsworth, 2007); Barbara Bloom, Barbara Owen, and

Stephanie Covington, "Gender-Responsive Strategies: Research, Practice, and Guiding Principles for Women Offenders" (Washington: National Institute of Corrections, 2003); Meda Chesney-Lind and Joycelyn Pollock, "Women's Prisons: Equality with a Vengeance," in *Women, Law, and Social Control*, ed. Alida Merlo and Joycelyn Pollock (Boston: Allyn and Bacon, 1995).

CHAPTER 4   GLADSTONE LODGE:
            HAVEN FOR THE CHEMICALLY
            DEPENDENT

1. The tenth step in the original twelve-step program of Alcoholics Anonymous reads "[We] continued to take personal inventory and when we were wrong promptly admitted it" (Alcoholics Anonymous World Services, "The Twelve Steps of Alcoholics Anonymous," revised August 2016, accessed October 2, 2016, http://www.aa.org/assets/en_US/smf-121_en.pdf).

2. At Gladstone Lodge, the staff used "addiction" generically to refer to all forms of chemical dependency. However, they often referred to individuals as either alcoholics or (drug) addicts and to recovery as being sober or being clean. As explained in chapter 2, I use terms such as "addict" and "sober" generically to include alcohol and other drugs.

3. Carl E. Thune, "Alcoholism and the Archetypal Past: A Phenomenological Perspective on Alcoholics Anonymous," *Journal of Studies on Alcohol* 38, no. 1 (1977): 75–88; Harrison M. Trice and Paul Michael Roman, "Delabeling, Relabeling and Alcoholics Anonymous," *Social Problems* 17, no. 4 (1970).

4. Teresa Gowan and Sarah Whetstone, "Making the Criminal Addict: Subjectivity and Social Control in a Strong-Arm Rehab," *Punishment and Society* 14, no. 1 (2012): 69–93; Jill McCorkel, *Breaking Women: Gender, Race, and the New Politics of Imprisonment* (New York: New York University Press, 2013); Rebecca Tiger, *Judging Addicts: Drug Courts and Coercion in the Justice System* (New York: New York University Press, 2012).

5. Critics of AA/NA make the same points, condemning the organizations' denial of agency, conformist ideals, and the stigma of a permanent addict label. See Lance Dodes and Zachary Dodes, *The Sober Truth: Debunking the Bad Science Behind 12-Step Programs and the Rehab Industry* (Boston: Beacon, 2014); Stanton Peele, *Diseasing of America: Addiction Treatment out of Control* (New York: Lexington, 1995).

6. In AA, the only criterion for participation is a "sincere desire to stop drinking." Lodge staff members wanted to model their program after AA, so it was important that all clients met that criterion. Because the police department's referral system did not depend on a diagnosis of chemical dependency, the Lodge had to find a work-around for Elsa.

7. Alcoholics Anonymous World Services, "The Twelve Steps of Alcoholics Anonymous."

8. Gladstone Lodge also has "contracts," in which clients agree not to do something again. This is common terminology in the field, but it had different ideological uses at WTS.

9. State funds cannot be used to promote religion, but the Lodge's "higher power" explanation for eschewing public funding is not very convincing because state authorities do not always consider twelve-step programs to be religious. The state agency that regulates and funds alternative-to-incarceration (ATI) programs requires them to be secular. Nevertheless, WTS had voluntary spiritual groups and expected clients to attend NA meetings. Meanwhile, the Lodge often noted that the steps' "higher power" could be a secular entity. Criminal justice systems

regularly sentence people to participate in twelve-step groups, even though some courts have held that these groups are religious and thus participation in them cannot be required (see, for example, the decisions in two US Court of Appeals cases, *Kerr v. Farrey* in the Seventh Circuit in 1996, and *Warner v. Orange County Dept. of Probation*, in the Second Circuit in 1997). I never found confirmation of the rule preventing counselors from disclosing their own experiences.

10. The only counselor in the women's program who was not a former addict had a husband who was, and she was active in twelve-step groups for family members like Al-Anon.

11. I calculated this using the National Addiction and HIV Data Archive Program, "Treatment Episode Data Set—Admissions (TEDS-A)—Concatenated 1992 to 2012," accessed November 4, 2013, http://www.icpsr.umich.edu/icpsrweb/NAHDAP/studies/25221.

12. The fourth step is "make a searching and fearless moral inventory of ourselves," and the fifth is "admitted to God, to ourselves and to another human being the exact nature of our wrongs" (Alcoholics Anonymous World Services, "The Twelve Steps of Alcoholics Anonymous").

13. Michael Omi and Howard Winant. *Racial Formation in the United States* (New York: Routledge, 1994).

14. Norman Kent Denzin, *The Alcoholic Society: Addiction and Recovery of the Self* (New Brunswick, NJ: Transaction, 1993); Leslie Irvine, *Codependent Forevermore: The Invention of Self in a Twelve Step Group* (Chicago: University of Chicago Press, 1999); Darin Weinberg, *Of Others Inside: Insanity, Addiction, and Belonging in America* (Philadelphia: Temple University Press, 2005).

15. For one prominent example, see Peele, *Diseasing of America*.

16. Mariana Valverde has argued the same thing about AA's use of storytelling and the flexibility rather than dogmatism of its methods (*Diseases of the Will: Alcohol and the Dilemmas of Freedom* [New York: Cambridge University Press, 1998]).

17. Weinberg, *Of Others Inside,* 74. Interestingly Weinberg studied inpatient and out-patient programs for marginalized and homeless people, but he found even there this effort to distance the self from the addiction. However, his research sites were not penal rehab programs, which may explain why they were not as stigmatizing as criminal justice programs.

18. Erving Goffman, *Stigma: Notes on the Management of Spoiled Identity* (New York: Simon and Schuster, 1963).

19. Once a week the entire staff of Gladstone Lodge met at lunch and one staff member would tell his or her story. This was seen as the staff's AA/NA meeting.

20. Michel Foucault, *Discipline and Punish: The Birth of the Prison*, trans. Alan Sheridan (New York: Vintage, 1977).

21. Books and magazines are banned because clients are not allowed to have any reading material that is not provided by the program. Only recovery literature and selected newspapers are provided.

22. Kristina Wandzilak and Constance Curry, *The Lost Years: Surviving a Mother and Daughter's Worst Nightmare* (Santa Monica, CA: Jeffers, 2006).

23. The theologian Reinhold Niebuhr is credited with originating the prayer in the 1930s, which was later popularized by AA. See Fred R. Shapiro, "Who Wrote the Serenity Prayer," *Chronicle of Higher Education,* April 28, 2014, accessed October 5, 2016, http://chronicle.com/article/Who-Wrote-the-Serenity-Prayer-/146159/. The version I quote from is the one recited at the Lodge and WTS.

CHAPTER 5 GLADSTONE LODGE: LEARNING TO LIVE
      SOBER

1. Mariana Valverde, *Diseases of the Will: Alcohol and the Dilemmas of Freedom* (New York: Cambridge University Press, 1998), 5.
2. Alcoholics Anonymous World Services, "The Twelve Steps of Alcoholics Anonymous," revised August 2016, accessed October 2, 2016, http://www.aa.org/assets/en_US/smf-121_en.pdf.
3. Alcoholics Anonymous World Services, *Alcoholics Anonymous: The Story of How Many Thousands of Men and Women Have Recovered from Alcoholism*, 4th ed. (New York: Alcoholics Anonymous World Services, 2001), 62.
4. Trysh Travis, *The Language of the Heart: A Cultural History of the Recovery Movement from Alcoholics Anonymous to Oprah Winfrey* (Chapel Hill: University of North Carolina Press, 2009), 62 and 65.
5. Ibid. See also Nancy Campbell and Elizabeth Ettorre, *Gendering Addiction: The Politics of Drug Treatment in a Neurochemical World* (New York: Palgrave Macmillan, 2011); John Steadman Rice, *A Disease of One's Own: Psychotherapy, Addiction, and the Emergence of Co-Dependency* (New Brunswick, NJ: Transaction, 1996).
6. Campbell and Ettore, *Gendering Addiction*.
7. In keeping with AA's and NA's Christian roots, a few staff members recited the Lord's Prayer after group meetings in addition to the standard Serenity Prayer.
8. The men were also clearly smoking during their walk.
9. Norman Kent Denzin, *The Alcoholic Society: Addiction and Recovery of the Self* (New Brunswick, NJ: Transaction, 1993); Leslie Irvine, *Codependent Forevermore: The Invention of Self in a Twelve Step Group* (Chicago: University of Chicago Press, 1999).
10. Harrison M. Trice and Paul Michael Roman, "Delabeling, Relabeling, and Alcoholics Anonymous," *Social Problems* 17, no. 4 (1970).
11. I think this list was taken from Sarah Ban Breathnach, *The Simple Abundance Journal of Gratitude* (New York: Warner Books, 1996).
12. Lynne Haney, *Offending Women: Gender, Punishment, and the Regulation of Desire* (Berkeley: University of California Press, 2010).
13. Patrick Biernacki, *Pathways from Heroin Addiction: Recovery without Treatment* (Philadelphia: Temple University Press, 1986).

CONCLUSION

1. Nancy Fraser, *Unruly Practices: Power, Discourse, and Gender in Contemporary Social Theory* (Minneapolis: University of Minnesota Press, 1989), 145.
2. Loïc Wacquant, "Deadly Symbiosis: When Ghetto and Prison Meet and Merge," in *Mass Imprisonment*, ed. David Garland (London: Sage, 2001).
3. Nikolas Rose, *Powers of Freedom. Reframing Political Thought* (Cambridge: Cambridge University Press, 1999). See also Barbara Cruikshank, *The Will to Empower: Democratic Citizens and Other Subjects* (Ithaca, NY: Cornell University Press, 1999).
4. Nikolas Rose, "Government and Control," *British Journal of Criminology* 40, no. 2 (2000): 335.
5. Lynne Haney, *Offending Women: Gender, Punishment, and the Regulation of Desire* (Berkeley: University of California Press, 2010).
6. David Garland, *The Culture of Control: Crime and Social Order in Contemporary Society* (Chicago: University of Chicago Press, 2001).
7. Rose, "Government and Control."
8. Wacquant, "Deadly Symbiosis," 103.
9. Katherine Beckett, Kris Nyrop, Lori Pfingst, and Melissa Bowen, "Drug Use, Drug Possession Arrests, and the Question of Race: Lessons from Seattle," *Social Problems* 52, no. 3 (2005); Alexes Harris, Heather Evans, and Katherine Beckett, "Courtesy

Stigma and Monetary Sanctions toward a Socio-Cultural Theory of Punishment," *American Sociological Review* 76, no. 2 (2011).

10. Devah Pager, "The Mark of a Criminal Record," *American Journal of Sociology* 108, no. 5 (2003).

11. Prominent examples include Teresa Gowan and Sarah Whetstone, "Making the Criminal Addict: Subjectivity and Social Control in a Strong-Arm Rehab," *Punishment and Society* 14, no. 1 (2012); Haney, *Offending Women*; Kerwin Kaye, "Drug Courts and the Treatment of Addiction: Therapeutic Jurisprudence and Neoliberal Governance" (PhD diss., New York University, 2010); Jill McCorkel, *Breaking Women: Gender, Race, and the New Politics of Imprisonment* (New York: New York University Press, 2013).

12. Substance Abuse and Mental Health Services Administration, "Facilities Offering Special Programs or Groups for Women: 2005," *DASIS Report*, issue 6 (2005), accessed October 8, 2016, http://archive.samhsa.gov/data/2k6/womenTx/womenTX.htm.

13. Christine E. Grella, "From Generic to Gender-Responsive Treatment: Changes in Social Policies, Treatment Services, and Outcomes of Women in Substance Abuse Treatment," *Journal of Psychoactive Drugs* 40, supplement 5 (2008): 333.

14. Lisa Maher, *Sexed Work: Gender, Race, and Resistance in a Brooklyn Drug Market* (New York: Oxford University Press, 1997).

15. Haney, *Offending Women*.

16. Jill McCorkel, "Criminally Dependent? Gender, Punishment, and the Rhetoric of Welfare Reform," *Social Politics* 11, no. 3 (2004).

17. On weak ego boundaries, see Jessica J. B. Wyse, "Rehabilitating Criminal Selves: Gendered Strategies in Community Corrections," *Gender and Society* 27, no. 2 (2013). On self-esteem, see Sara Goodkind, "'You Can Be Anything You Want, but You Have to Believe It': Commercialized Feminism in Gender Specific Programs for Girls," *Signs* 34, no. 2 (2009); Miranda March, "Rubrics of Rehabilitation: Gendered Narratives of Selfhood in Court Mandated Treatment Facilities" (PhD diss., New York University, 2009).

18. Patricia Hill Collins, *Black Feminist Thought: Knowledge, Consciousness, and the Politics of Empowerment*, 2nd ed. (New York: Routledge, 2000), 69.

19. Cruikshank, *The Will to Empower*.

20. Arlie Hochschild and Anne Machung, *The Second Shift: Working Families and the Revolution at Home*, 2nd ed. (New York: Penguin, 2012).

21. Lynne Haney found the same thing: staff members would tell women who made arguments about social constraints that "the system is in your head" (*Offending Women*, 166).

22. For example, see Institute of Medicine, *Bridging the Gap between Practice and Research: Forging Partnerships with Community-Based Drug and Alcohol Treatment* (Washington: National Academies Press, 1998). Eleven and fourteen years later the following reports made similar critiques and recommendations: Dennis McCarthy, K. John McConnell, and Laura A. Schmidt, "Policies for the Treatment of Alcohol and Drug Use Disorders: A Research Agenda for 2010–2015 (Highlights)" (Princeton, NJ: Robert Wood Johnson Foundation, 2009), accessed September 30, 2016, http://www.rwjf.org/content/dam/farm/reports/reports/2009/rwjf46848; National Center on Addiction and Substance Abuse, *Addiction Medicine: Closing the Gap between Science and Practice* (New York: Columbia University, 2012), downloaded

October 8, 2016, http://www.centeronaddiction.org/addiction-research/reports/ addiction-medicine.

METHODOLOGICAL APPENDIX

1. Michael Burawoy, *The Extended Case Method: Four Countries, Four Decades, Four Great Transformations, and One Theoretical Tradition* (Berkeley: University of California Press, 2009).
2. Michael Burawoy, "The Extended Case Method," *Sociological Theory* 16, no. 1 (1998): 5.
3. Shamus Khan and Colin Jerolmack, "Saying Meritocracy and Doing Privilege," *Sociological Quarterly* 54, no. 1 (2013).
4. I used state and federal databases as well as general search engines.

BIBLIOGRAPHY

Adams, Julia, and Tasleem Padamsee. "Signs and Regimes: Rereading Feminist Work on Welfare States." *Social Politics* 8, no. 1 (2001): 1–23.

Alcoholics Anonymous World Services. *Alcoholics Anonymous: The Story of How Many Thousands of Men and Women Have Recovered from Alcoholism.* 4th ed. New York: Alcoholics Anonymous World Services, 2001.

Alexander, Michelle. *The New Jim Crow: Mass Incarceration in the Age of Colorblindness.* New York: New Press, 2012.

Alexander, Ruth M. *The "Girl Problem": Female Sexual Delinquency in New York 1900–1930.* Ithaca, NY: Cornell University Press, 1995.

Anderson, Tammy L. *Neither Villain nor Victim: Empowerment and Agency among Women Substance Abusers.* New Brunswick, NJ: Rutgers University Press, 2008.

Becker, Howard. *Outsiders: Studies in the Sociology of Deviance.* New York: Free Press, 1963.

Beckett, Katherine. *Making Crime Pay: Law and Order in Contemporary American Politics.* New York: Oxford University Press, 1999.

———, and Naomi Murakawa. "Mapping the Shadow Carceral State: Toward an Institutionally Capacious Approach to Punishment." *Theoretical Criminology* 16, no. 2 (2012): 221-44.

Beckett, Katherine, Kris Nyrop, Lori Pfingst, and Melissa Bowen. "Drug Use, Drug Possession Arrests, and the Question of Race: Lessons from Seattle." *Social Problems* 52, no. 3 (2005): 419–41.

Beckett, Katherine, and Bruce Western. "Governing Social Marginality: Welfare, Incarceration, and the Transformation of State Policy." In *Mass Imprisonment: Social Causes and Consequences,* edited by David Garland, 35-5-. London: Sage, 2001.

Belknap, Joanne. *The Invisible Woman: Gender, Crime, and Justice.* 3rd ed. Belmont, CA: Wadsworth, 2007.

Biernacki, Patrick. *Pathways from Heroin Addiction: Recovery without Treatment.* Philadelphia: Temple University Press, 1986.

Bloom, Barbara, Barbara Owen, and Stephanie Covington. "Gender-Responsive Strategies: Research, Practice, and Guiding Principles for Women Offenders." Washington: National Institute of Corrections, 2003.

Bouffard, Jeff, and Faye Taxman. "Looking Inside the 'Black Box' of Drug Court Treatment Services Using Direct Observations." *Journal of Drug Issues* 34, no. 1 (2004): 195–218.

Bourdieu, Pierre. *Outline of a Theory of Practice.* Translated by Richard Nice. Cambridge: Cambridge University Press, 1977.

Brady, Thomas M., and Olivia S. Ashley. "Women in Substance Abuse Treatment: Results from the Alcohol and Drug Services Study (ADSS)." Rockville, MD: Substance Abuse and Mental Health Service Administration, 2005.

Britton, Dana M. *At Work in the Iron Cage: The Prison as a Gendered Organization.* New York: New York University Press, 2003.

Burawoy, Michael. "The Extended Case Method." *Sociological Theory* 16, no. 1 (1998): 4-33.

———. *The Extended Case Method:* Four Countries, Four Decades, Four Great Transformations, and One Theoretical Tradition. Berkeley: University of California Press, 2009.

Bureau of Justice Assistance. "Residential Substance Abuse Treatment for State Prisoners (RSAT) Program." Washington: Bureau of Justice Assistance, April 2005. Accessed October 2, 2016. https://www.ncjrs.gov/pdffiles1/bja/206269.pdf.

Campbell, Nancy. *Discovering Addiction: The Science and Politics of Substance Abuse Research.* Ann Arbor: University of Michigan Press, 2007.

———. *Using Women: Gender, Drug Policy, and Social Justice.* New York: Routledge, 2000.

———and Elizabeth Ettorre. *Gendering Addiction: The Politics of Drug Treatment in a Neurochemical World.* New York: Palgrave Macmillan, 2011.

Chasnoff, Ira J., Harvey J. Landress, and Mark E. Barrett. "The Prevalence of Illicit-Drug or Alcohol Use during Pregnancy and Discrepancies in Mandatory Reporting in Pinellas County, Florida." *New England Journal of Medicine* 322, no. 17 (1990): 1202–6.

Chesney-Lind, Meda. "Girls' Crime and Woman's Place: Toward a Feminist Model of Female Delinquency." *Crime and Delinquency* 35, no. 1 (1989): 5–29.

———and Joycelyn Pollock. "Women's Prisons: Equality with a Vengeance." In *Women, Law, and Social Control,* edited by Alida Merlo and Joycelyn Pollock, 155–76. Boston: Allyn and Bacon, 1995.

Cloud, William, and Robert Granfield. "Conceptualizing Recovery Capital: Expansion of a Theoretical Construct." *Substance Use and Misuse* 43, nos. 12-13 (2008): 1971–86.

———. "Natural Recovery from Substance Dependency." *Journal of Social Work Practice in the Addictions* 1, no. 1 (2001): 83–104.

Collins, Patricia Hill. *Black Feminist Thought: Knowledge, Consciousness, and the Politics of Empowerment.* 2nd ed. New York: Routledge, 2000.

Conrad, Peter, and Joseph Schneider. *Deviance and Medicalization: From Badness to Sickness.* Philadelphia: Temple University Press, 1992.

Courtwright, David T. *Dark Paradise: A History of Opiate Addiction in America.* Enlarged ed. Cambridge, MA: Harvard University Press, 2001.

Cruikshank, Barbara. *The Will to Empower: Democratic Citizens and Other Subjects.* Ithaca, NY: Cornell University Press, 1999.

DeLeon, George. *The Therapeutic Community: Theory, Model, and Method.* New York: Springer, 2000.

Delpit, Lisa. "The Silenced Dialogue: Power and Pedagogy in Educating Other People's Children." *Harvard Educational Review* 58, no. 3 (1988): 280–98.

Denzin, Norman Kent. *The Alcoholic Society: Addiction and Recovery of the Self.* New Brunswick, NJ: Transaction, 1993.

Dodes, Lance, and Zachary Dodes. *The Sober Truth: Debunking the Bad Science Behind 12-Step Programs and the Rehab Industry.* Boston: Beacon, 2014.

Edin, Kathryn, and Maria Kefalas. *Promises I Can Keep: Why Poor Women Put Motherhood before Marriage.* Berkeley: University of California Press, 2005.

Enos, Sandra. *Mothering from the Inside: Parenting in a Women's Prison.* Albany: State University of New York Press, 2001.

Erikson, Kai. *Wayward Puritans: A Study in the Sociology of Deviance.* Rev. ed. Boston: Pearson/Allyn and Bacon, 2005.

Fairbanks, Robert P. *How It Works: Recovering Citizens in Post-Welfare Philadelphia.* Chicago: University of Chicago Press, 2009.

Feeley, Malcolm, and Jonathan Simon. "The New Penology: Notes on the Emerging Strategy of Corrections and Its Implications." *Criminology* 30, no. 4 (1992): 449–70.

Ferraro, Kathleen J., and Angela M. Moe. "Mothering, Crime, and Incarceration." *Journal of Contemporary Ethnography* 32, no. 1 (2003): 9–40.

Flavin, Jeanne. "Of Punishment and Parenthood: Family-Based Social Control and the Sentencing of Black Drug Offenders." *Gender and Society* 15, no. 4 (2001): 611–33.

———. *Our Bodies, Our Crimes: The Policing of Women's Reproduction in America.* New York: New York University Press, 2009.

———and Lynn M. Paltrow. "Punishing Pregnant Drug-Using Women: Defying Law, Medicine, and Common Sense." *Journal of Addictive Diseases* 29, no. 2 (2010): 231–44.

Fletcher, Anne. *Inside Rehab: The Surprising Truth about Addiction Treatment—and How to Get Help That Works.* New York: Viking, 2013.

Foucault, Michel. *Discipline and Punish: The Birth of the Prison.* Translated by Alan Sheridan. New York: Vintage, 1977.

———. "Governmentality." In *The Foucault Effect: Studies in Governmentality,* edited by Graham Burchell, Colin Gordon, and Peter Miller, 87-104. Chicago: University of Chicago Press, 1991.

———. *The History of Sexuality.* Vol. 3: *The Care of the Self.* Translated by Robert Hurley. New York: Vintage, 1986.

Frank, Deborah A., Marilyn Augustyn, Wanda Grant Knight, Tripler Pell, and Barry Zuckerman. "Growth, Development, and Behavior in Early Childhood Following Prenatal Cocaine Exposure: A Systematic Review." *Journal of the American Medical Association* 285, no. 12 (2001): 1613–25.

Fraser, Nancy. *Unruly Practices: Power, Discourse, and Gender in Contemporary Social Theory.* Minneapolis: University of Minnesota Press, 1989.

———, and Linda Gordon. "A Genealogy of Dependency: Tracing a Keyword of the U.S. Welfare State." In *Justice Interruptus,* edited by Nancy Fraser, 121-49. New York: Routledge, 1997.

Gaines, Kevin K. *Uplifting the Race: Black Leadership, Politics, and Culture in the Twentieth Century.* Chapel Hill: University of North Carolina Press, 1996.

Garfinkel, Harold. "Conditions of Successful Degradation Ceremonies." *American Journal of Sociology* 61, no. 5 (1956): 420–24.

Garland, David. *The Culture of Control: Crime and Social Order in Contemporary Society.* Chicago: University of Chicago Press, 2001.

———. "Introduction: The Meaning of Mass Imprisonment." In *Mass Imprisonment: Social Causes and Consequences,* edited by David Garland, 1-3. London: Sage, 2001.

———. *Punishment and Modern Society: A Study in Social Theory.* Chicago: University of Chicago Press, 1990.

———. *Punishment and Welfare: A History of Penal Strategies.* Aldershot, UK: Gower, 1985.

Glaze, Lauren E. "Correctional Populations in the United States, 2009." Washington: Bureau of Justice Statistics, December 2010. Accessed September 30, 2016. http://bjs.gov/content/pub/pdf/cpus09.pdf.

Goffman, Erving. *Asylums: Essays on the Social Situation of Mental Patients and Other Inmates.* New York: Anchor, 1961.

———. *The Presentation of Self in Everyday Life.* New York: Anchor, 1959.

———. *Stigma: Notes on the Management of Spoiled Identity.* New York: Simon and Schuster, 1963. Goldkamp, John S., Michael D. White, and Jennifer B. Robinson. "Do Drug

Courts Work? Getting Inside the Drug Court Black Box." *Journal of Drug Issues* 31, no. 1 (2001): 27–72.

Gomez, Laura. *Misconceiving Mothers: Legislators, Prosecutors, and the Politics of Prenatal Drug Exposure.* Philadelphia: Temple University Press, 1997.

Goodkind, Sara. "'You Can Be Anything You Want, but You Have to Believe It': Commercialized Feminism in Gender Specific Programs for Girls." *Signs* 34, no. 2 (2009): 397–422.

Gottschalk, Marie. *The Shadow Welfare State: Labor, Business, and the Politics of Health-Care in the United States.* Ithaca, NY: Cornell University Press, 2000.

Gowan, Teresa. *Hobos, Hustlers, and Backsliders: Homeless in San Francisco.* Minneapolis: University of Minnesota Press, 2010.

————and Sarah Whetstone. "Making the Criminal Addict: Subjectivity and Social Control in a Strong-Arm Rehab." *Punishment and Society* 14, no. 1 (2012): 69–93.

Grella, Christine E. "From Generic to Gender-Responsive Treatment: Changes in Social Policies, Treatment Services, and Outcomes of Women in Substance Abuse Treatment." *Journal of Psychoactive Drugs* 40, supplement 5 (2008): 327–43.

Gusfield, Joseph R. *Symbolic Crusade: Status Politics and the American Temperance Movement.* 2nd ed. Urbana: University of Illinois Press, 1986.

Hackett, Colleen. "Transformative Visions: Governing through Alternative Practices and Therapeutic Interventions at a Women's Reentry Center." *Feminist Criminology* 8, no. 3 (2013): 221–42.

Haney, Lynne. "Gender, Welfare, and States of Punishment." *Social Politics* 11, no. 3 (2004): 333–62.

————. *Offending Women: Gender, Punishment, and the Regulation of Desire.* Berkeley: University of California Press, 2010.

Hannah-Moffat, Kelly. "Assembling Risk and the Restructuring of Penal Control." *British Journal of Criminology* 46 (2006): 438–54.

————. "Criminogenic Needs and the Transformative Risk Subject: Hybridizations of Risk/Need in Penality." *Punishment and Society* 7, no. 1 (2005): 29–51.

————. "Feminine Fortresses: Women-Centered Prisons?" *Prison Journal* 75, no. 2 (1995): 71–94.

————. "Losing Ground: Gendered Knowledges, Parole Risk, and Responsibility." *Social Politics* 11, no. 3 (2004): 363–85.

————. "Moral Agent or Actuarial Subject: Risk and Canadian Women's Imprisonment." *Theoretical Criminology* 3, no. 1 (1999): 71–94.

————. "Prisons That Empower: Neo-Liberal Governance in Canadian Women's Prisons." *British Journal of Criminology* 40, no. 3 (2000): 510–31.

Harlow, Caroline Wolf. "Prior Abuse Reported by Inmates and Probationers." Washington: Bureau of Justice Statistics, April 1999. Accessed October 2, 2016. https://www.prearesourcecenter.org/sites/default/files/library/priorabusereportedbyinmatesandprobationers.pdf.

Harris, Alexes, Heather Evans, and Katherine Beckett. "Courtesy Stigma and Monetary Sanctions toward a Socio-Cultural Theory of Punishment." *American Sociological Review* 76, no. 2 (2011): 234–64.

Hays, Sharon. *The Cultural Contradictions of Motherhood.* New Haven, CT: Yale University Press, 1998.

————. *Flat Broke with Children: Women in the Age of Welfare Reform.* New York: Oxford University Press, 2004.

Hochschild, Arlie. *The Commercialization of Intimate Life: Notes from Home and Work.* Berkeley: University of California Press, 2003.

———and Anne Machung. *The Second Shift: Working Families and the Revolution at Home.* 2nd ed. New York: Penguin, 2012.

Humphries, Drew. *Crack Mothers: Pregnancy, Drugs, and the Media.* Columbus: Ohio State University Press, 1999.

Institute of Medicine, *Bridging the Gap between Practice and Research: Forging Partnerships with Community-Based Drug and Alcohol Treatment* (Washington: National Academies Press, 1998).

Irvine, Leslie. *Codependent Forevermore: The Invention of Self in a Twelve Step Group.* Chicago: University of Chicago Press, 1999.

Kaeble, Danielle, Lauren Glaze, Anastasios Tsoutis, and Todd Minton. "Correctional Populations in the United States, 2014." Washington: Bureau of Justice Statistics, January 21, 2016. Accessed September 2016. http://www.bjs.gov/content/pub/pdf/cpus14.pdf.

Kaye, Kerwin. "Drug Courts and the Treatment of Addiction: Therapeutic Jurisprudence and Neoliberal Governance." PhD diss., New York University, 2010.

———. "Rehabilitating the 'Drugs Lifestyle': Criminal Justice, Social Control, and the Cultivation of Agency." *Ethnography* 14, no. 2 (2013): 207–32.

Keire, Mara L. "Dope Fiends and Degenerates: The Gendering of Addiction in the Early Twentieth Century." *Journal of Social History* 31, no. 4 (1998): 809–22.

Khan, Shamus, and Colin Jerolmack. "Saying Meritocracy and Doing Privilege." *Sociological Quarterly* 54, no. 1 (2013): 9–19.

Kohler-Hausmann, Issa. "Misdemeanor Justice: Control without Conviction." *American Journal of Sociology* 119, no. 2 (2013): 351–93.

Kruttschnitt, Candace, and Rosemary Gartner. *Marking Time in the Golden State: Women's Imprisonment in California.* Cambridge: Cambridge University Press, 2005.

———and Amy Miller. "Doing Her Own Time? Women's Responses to Prison in the Context of the Old and the New Penology." *Criminology* 38, no. 3 (2000): 681–717.

Levine, Harry G. "The Discovery of Addiction: Changing Conceptions of Habitual Drunkenness in America." *Journal of Studies on Alcohol* 39, no. 1 (1978): 143-74.

Maher, Lisa. *Sexed Work: Gender, Race, and Resistance in a Brooklyn Drug Market.* New York: Oxford University Press, 1997.

Manza, Jeff, and Christopher Uggen. *Locked Out: Felon Disenfranchisement and American Democracy.* New York: Oxford University Press, 2008.

March, Miranda. "Rubrics of Rehabilitation: Gendered Narratives of Selfhood in Court Mandated Treatment Facilities." PhD diss., New York University, 2009. Mauer, Marc. "The Causes and Consequences of Prison Growth in the United States." *Punishment and Society* 3, no. 1 (2001): 9–20.

———. "Our Compassion for Drug Users Should Not Be Determined by Race." *Guardian,* January 7, 2016.

McCarty, Dennis, K. John McConnell, and Laura A. Schmidt. "Policies for the Treatment of Alcohol and Drug Use Disorders: A Research Agenda for 2010–2015 (Highlights)." Princeton, NJ: Robert Wood Johnson Foundation, October 2009. Accessed September 30, 2016. http://www.rwjf.org/content/dam/farm/reports/reports/2009/rwjf46848.

McCorkel, Jill. *Breaking Women: Gender, Race, and the New Politics of Imprisonment.* New York: New York University Press, 2013.

———. "Criminally Dependent? Gender, Punishment, and the Rhetoric of Welfare Reform." *Social Politics* 11, no. 3 (2004): 386–410.

———. "Embodied Surveillance and the Gendering of Punishment." *Journal of Contemporary Ethnography* 32, no. 1 (2003): 41–76.

McDaniels-Wilson, Cathy, and Joanne Belknap. "The Extensive Sexual Violation and Sexual Abuse Histories of Incarcerated Women." *Violence Against Women* 14, no. 10 (2008): 1090–127.

McGee, Micki. *Self-Help, Inc.: Makeover Culture in American Life.* New York: Oxford University Press, 2005.

McKim, Allison. "'Getting Gut-Level': Punishment, Gender, and Therapeutic Governance." *Gender and Society* 22, no. 3 (2008): 303–23.

———. "Roxanne's Dress: Governing Gender and Marginality through Addiction Treatment." *Signs* 39, no. 2 (2014): 433–58.

Miller, Reuben Jonathan. "Devolving the Carceral State: Race, Prisoner Reentry, and the Micro-Politics of Urban Poverty Management." *Punishment and Society* 16, no. 3 (2014): 305–35.

Mink, Gwendolyn. "The Lady and the Tramp: Gender, Race, and the Origins of the American Welfare State." In *Women, the State, and Welfare,* edited by Linda Gordon, 92–122. Madison: University of Wisconsin Press, 1990.

Musto, David. *The American Disease: Origins of Narcotics Control.* 3rd ed. New York: Oxford University Press, 1999.

National Center on Addiction and Substance Abuse. *Addiction Medicine: Closing the Gap between Science and Practice.* New York: Columbia University, 2012. Downloaded October 8, 2016. http://www.centeronaddiction.org/addiction-research/reports/addiction-medicine.

O'Connor, Julia S., Ann Shola Orloff, and Sheila Shaver. *States, Markets, Families: Gender, Liberalism, and Social Policy in Australia, Canada, Great Britain, and the United States.* New York: Cambridge University Press, 1999.

Odem, Mary. *Delinquent Daughters: Protecting and Policing Adolescent Female Sexuality in the United States, 1885–1920.* Chapel Hill: University of North Carolina Press, 1995.

Omi, Michael, and Howard Winant. *Racial Formation in the United States.* New York: Routledge, 1994.

Pager, Devah. "The Mark of a Criminal Record." *American Journal of Sociology* 108, no. 5 (2003): 937–75.

———. *Marked: Race, Crime, and Finding Work in an Era of Mass Incarceration.* Chicago: University of Chicago Press, 2007.

Paltrow, Lynn M., and Jeanne Flavin. "Arrests of and Forced Interventions on Pregnant Women in the United States, 1973–2005: Implications for Women's Legal Status and Public Health." *Journal of Health Politics, Policy and Law* 38, no. 2 (2013): 299–343.

Peele, Stanton. *Diseasing of America: Addiction Treatment out of Control.* New York: Lexington, 1995.

Phelps, Michelle S. "Rehabilitation in the Punitive Era: The Gap between Rhetoric and Reality in US Prison Programs." *Law and Society Review* 45, no. 1 (2011): 33–68.

Pollack, Shoshana. "'I'm Just Not Good in Relationships': Victimization Discourses and the Gender Regulation of Criminalized Women." *Feminist Criminology* 2 (2007): 158–74.

Porter, Rachel, Sophia Lee, and Mary Lutz. "Balancing Treatment and Punishment: Alternatives to Incarceration in New York City." New York: Vera Institute for Justice, 2002.

Rafter, Nicole Hahn. *Partial Justice: Women, Prisons, and Social Control.* New Brunswick, NJ: Transaction, 1995.

Reich, Jennifer. *Fixing Families: Parents, Power, and the Child Welfare System.* New York: Routledge, 2005.

Reinarman, Craig, and Harold Levine. *Crack in America: Demon Drugs and Social Justice.* Berkeley: University of California Press, 1997.

Rice, John Steadman. *A Disease of One's Own: Psychotherapy, Addiction, and the Emergence of Co-Dependency.* New Brunswick, NJ: Transaction, 1996.

Richie, Beth E. *Arrested Justice: Black Women, Violence, and America's Prison Nation.* New York: New York University Press, 2012.

Roberts, Dorothy. *Killing the Black Body: Race, Reproduction, and the Meaning of Liberty.* New York: Vintage, 1998.

————. "Motherhood and Crime." *Social Text* 42 (Spring 1995): 99–123.

————. "Punishing Drug Addicts Who Have Babies: Women of Color, Equality, and the Right of Privacy." *Harvard Law Review* 104, no. 7 (1990): 1419-82.

————. "Racism and Patriarchy in the Meaning of Motherhood." *American University Journal of Gender and Law* 1, no.1 (1993): 1-38.

————. *Shattered Bonds: The Color of Child Welfare.* New York: Basic Civitas Books, 2002.

Robinson, Gwen. "Late-Modern Rehabilitation: The Evolution of a Penal Strategy." *Punishment and Society* 10, no. 4 (2008): 429-45.

Rose, Nikolas. *Governing the Soul: The Shaping of the Private Self.* 2nd ed. New York: Free Association, 1999.

————. "Government and Control." *British Journal of Criminology* 40, no. 2 (2000): 321–39.

————. *Powers of Freedom: Reframing Political Thought.* Cambridge: Cambridge University Press, 1999.

Rothman, David. *The Discovery of the Asylum: Social Order and Disorder in the New Republic.* Rev. ed. New York: Aldine de Gruyter, 2002.

Roychowdhury, Poulami. "Desire, Rights, Entitlements: Organizational Strategies in the War on Violence." *Signs* 41, no. 4 (2016): 793–820.

Schram, Sanford. "In the Clinic: The Medicalization of Welfare." *Social Text* 18, no. 1 (2000): 81–107.

Sentencing Project. "Fact Sheet: Trends in U.S. Corrections." Washington: Sentencing Project, December 2015. Accessed September 30, 2016. http://sentencingproject.org/wp-content/uploads/2016/01/Trends-in-US-Corrections.pdf.

Sered, Susan Starr, and Maureen Norton-Hawk. *Can't Catch a Break: Gender, Jail, Drugs, and the Limits of Personal Responsibility.* Berkeley: University of California Press, 2014.

Simon, Jonathan. *Governing through Crime: How the War on Crime Transformed American Democracy and Created a Culture of Fear.* New York: Oxford University Press, 2007.

————. *Poor Discipline: Parole and the Social Control of the Underclass, 1890–1990.* Chicago: University of Chicago Press, 1993.

Stuart, Forrest. "From 'Rabble Management' to 'Recovery Management': Policing Homelessness in Marginal Urban Space." *Urban Studies* 51, no. 9 (2013): 1909-25.

Substance Abuse and Mental Health Services Administration. "Facilities Offering Special Programs or Groups for Women: 2005." *DASIS Report*, issue 6 (2005). Accessed October 8, 2016. http://archive.samhsa.gov/data/2k6/womenTx/womenTX.htm.

————. "National Expenditures for Mental Health Services and Substance Abuse Treatment, 1986–2009." Rockville, MD: Substance Abuse and Mental Health Services Administration, 2013. Accessed September 30, 2016. https://store.samhsa.gov/shin/content/SMA13-4740/SMA13-4740.pdf.

————. "National Survey of Substance Abuse Treatment Services (NSSATS): 2010: Data on Substance Abuse Treatment Facilities." Rockville, MD: Substance Abuse and

Mental Health Services Administration, September 2011. Accessed September 30, 2016. http://wwwdasis.samhsa.gov/10nssats/NSSATS2010Web.pdf.

———. "Participation in Self-Help Groups for Alcohol and Illicit Drug Use: 2006 and 2007." Rockville, MD: Substance Abuse and Mental Health Services Administration, December 30, 2008. Accessed September 30, 2016. https://www.orange-papers.org/OAS.SAMHSA.GOV—selfHelp.htm.

———. "The TEDS Report: Substance Abuse Treatment Admissions Referred by the Criminal Justice System." Rockville, MD: Substance Abuse and Mental Health Services Administration, 2009.

———. "Treatment Episode Data Set (TEDS): 2000–2010: National Admissions to Substance Abuse Treatment Services." Rockville, MD: Substance Abuse and Mental Health Services Administration, June 2012. Accessed September 30, 2016. http://wwwdasis.samhsa.gov/dasis2/teds_pubs/2010_teds_rpt_natl.pdf.

———. "Treatment Episode Data Set (TEDS): 2004-2014: National Admissions to Substance Abuse Treatment Services." Rockville, MD: Substance Abuse and Mental Health Services Administration, 2016. Accessed November 1, 2016. http://www.samhsa.gov/data/sites/default/files/2014_Treatment_Episode_Data_Set_National_Admissions_9_19_16.pdf.

Sykes, Gresham. *The Society of Captives: A Study of a Maximum Security Prison.* Princeton, NJ: Princeton University Press, 2007.

Taxman, Faye S., and Jeffrey Bouffard. "Treatment Inside the Drug Court: The Who, What, Where, and How of Treatment Services." *Substance Use and Misuse* 37, nos. 12-13 (2002): 1665-88.

Taxman, Faye S., Matthew L. Perdoni, and Lana D. Harrison. "Drug Treatment Services for Adult Offenders: The State of the State." *Journal of Substance Abuse Treatment* 32, no. 3 (2007): 239–54.

Thune, Carl E. "Alcoholism and the Archetypal Past: A Phenomenological Perspective on Alcoholics Anonymous." *Journal of Studies on Alcohol* 38, no. 1 (1977): 75–88.

Tiger, Rebecca. *Judging Addicts: Drug Courts and Coercion in the Justice System.* New York: New York University Press, 2012.

Travis, Trysh. *The Language of the Heart: A Cultural History of the Recovery Movement from Alcoholics Anonymous to Oprah Winfrey.* Chapel Hill: University of North Carolina Press, 2009.

Trice, Harrison M., and Paul Michael Roman. "Delabeling, Relabeling, and Alcoholics Anonymous." *Social Problems* 17, no. 4 (1970): 538-46.

Valverde, Mariana. *Diseases of the Will: Alcohol and the Dilemmas of Freedom.* New York: Cambridge University Press, 1998.

Wacquant, Loïc. "Deadly Symbiosis: When Ghetto and Prison Meet and Merge." In *Mass Imprisonment: Social Causes and Consequences,* edited by David Garland, 82-120. London: Sage, 2001.

———. *Punishing the Poor: The Neoliberal Government of Social Insecurity.* Durham, NC: Duke University Press, 2009.

Ward, Geoff. *The Black Child-Savers: Racial Democracy and American Juvenile Justice.* Chicago: University of Chicago Press, 2012.

Weinberg, Darin. *Of Others Inside: Insanity, Addiction, and Belonging in America.* Philadelphia: Temple University Press, 2005.

Weisner, Constance, and Robin Room. "Financing and Ideology in Alcohol Treatment." *Social Problems* 32, no. 2 (1984): 167–84.

West, Candace, and Don Zimmerman. "Doing Gender." *Gender and Society* 1, no. 2 (1987): 125–51.

Western, Bruce. *Punishment and Inequality in America*. New York: Russell Sage Foundation, 2007.

White, William L. *Slaying the Dragon: The History of Addiction Treatment and Recovery in America*. Bloomington, IL: Chestnut Health Systems, 1998.

Wiener, Carolyn. *The Politics of Alcoholism: Building an Arena around a Social Problem*. New Brunswick, NJ: Transaction, 1981.

Williams, Patricia. *The Alchemy of Race and Rights*. Cambridge, MA: Harvard University Press, 1991.

Wyse, Jessica J. B. "Rehabilitating Criminal Selves: Gendered Strategies in Community Corrections." *Gender and Society* 27, no. 2 (2013): 231–55.

Index

AA. *See* Alcoholics Anonymous

abortion, 1, 73, 85, 201n9

abscond, 22, 37, 42, 55, 58, 66, 81

abstinence from drugs/alcohol, 24, 49, 143, 172

abuse: child abuse, 99–100, 140, 199n21; domestic violence, 3, 40, 53, 91, 103, 137, 152–154, 157, 163, 166, 169, 170; incest, 84; rape/sexual violence, 49–50, 53, 73, 84, 91, 135, 140, 163, 199n21; rehab as solution, 4, 10, 40, 91, 158, 168–173

addict, use of term, 198n2, 203n2

addict identity, 97, 115–120, 143, 147

addiction: construction/definition of, 3, 5, 13, 24, 56, 57, 65, 72, 73, 74, 89, 99–101, 102, 104, 115, 125, 127–128, 153, 156, 158, 162, 172–173, 198n2; discourse, 4-5, 12–13, 15, 16, 51–53, 73, 75, 158, 169–171 (*see also* therapeutic techniques); disease concept, 3, 6, 23, 24, 25–26, 102, 121, 127–128, 129, 195n5; gendered form of, 75, 98, 135, 137, 158, 164, 165; governing through, 9–16, 158–173 (*see also* governing through addiction); label/ stigma, 115–121, 125, 161–163, 203n5, 204n17; language, 5, 25, 56; "men's," 132; moral aspect of, 117–119; narrowing of, 101–107; politics of, 134–136; politics of motherhood, 87–90; racialized, 16, 125; respectable, 139–141; self-knowledge, 76–81, 141 (*see also* therapeutic techniques); use

of term, 198n2. *See also* alcoholism; codependence/dependence; gender; governing through addiction; race/ ethnicity; self; socioeconomic class; treatment program

Adoption and Safe Families Act, 195n1

Adriana (Gladstone Lodge client), 28, 137, 162, 169

Affordable Care Act, 4, 172

African American women: child welfare policies, 14, 38; client treatment, 1, 30, 38, 46, 170; devaluation of mother- hood, 90; drug use, 52, 90; incar- ceration rate, 191n27; motherhood as form of resistance, 90; parental drug use, 14; perceptions of, 8, 38. *See also* gender; Gladstone Lodge; race/eth- nicity; Women's Treatment Services

agency, 65, 119, 128, 130, 131, 136, 164–165, 203n5

Al-Anon, 204n10

Alcoholics Anonymous (AA), 4, 28, 100, 129, 203nn5, 6; history, 25–26; and rehab workers, 23, 108–109; religious- like directive, 107, 205n7; Seren- ity Prayer, 124, 131, 204n23; social redemption, 144; telling one's story, 117, 204n16; twelve steps, 2, 34–35, 101–102, 130, 143, 201n9. *See also* "Big Book"; Narcotics Anonymous; Synanon; twelve-step program

alcoholism, 23, 25, 26, 28, 189n3, 195n5. *See also* addiction

About the Author

ALLISON MCKIM is an assistant professor of sociology at Bard College.

Available titles in the Critical Issues in Crime and Society series:

Laura S. Abrams and Diane J. Terry, *Life after Juvie: Young Men and Women on Desistence, Survival, and Becoming an Adult*

Tammy L. Anderson, ed., *Neither Villain nor Victim: Empowerment and Agency among Women Substance Abusers*

Scott A. Bonn, *Mass Deception: Moral Panic and the U.S. War on Iraq*

Mary Bosworth and Jeanne Flavin, eds., *Race, Gender, and Punishment: From Colonialism to the War on Terror*

Loretta Capeheart and Dragan Milovanovic, *Social Justice: Theories, Issues, and Movements*

Walter S. DeKeseredy and Martin D. Schwartz, *Dangerous Exits: Escaping Abusive Relationships in Rural America*

Patricia E. Erickson and Steven K. Erickson, *Crime, Punishment, and Mental Illness: Law and the Behavioral Sciences in Conflict*

Luis A. Fernandez, *Policing Dissent: Social Control and the Anti-Globalization Movement*

Mike King, *When Riot Cops are Not Enough: The Policing and Repression of Occupy Oakland*

Timothy R. Lauger, *Real Gangstas: Legitimacy, Reputation, and Violence in the Intergang Environment*

Michael J. Lynch, *Big Prisons, Big Dreams: Crime and the Failure of America's Penal System*

Allison McKim, *Addicted to Rehab: Race, Gender, and Drugs in the Era of Mass Incarceration*

Raymond J. Michalowski and Ronald C. Kramer, eds., *State-Corporate Crime: Wrongdoing at the Intersection of Business and Government*

Susan L. Miller, *Victims as Offenders: The Paradox of Women's Violence in Relationships*

Torin Monahan, *Surveillance in the Time of Insecurity*

Torin Monahan and Rodolfo D. Torres, eds., *Schools under Surveillance: Cultures of Control in Public Education*

Leslie Paik, *Discretionary Justice: Looking Inside a Juvenile Drug Court*

Anthony M. Platt, *The Child Savers: The Invention of Delinquency*, 40th anniversary edition with an introduction and critical commentaries compiled by Miroslava Chávez-García

Joshua M. Price, *Prison and Social Death*

Diana Rickard, *Sex Offenders, Stigma, and Social Control*

Jeffrey Ian Ross, ed., *The Globalization of Supermax Prisons*

Dawn L. Rothe and Christopher W. Mullins, eds., *State Crime, Current Perspectives*

Susan F. Sharp, *Hidden Victims: The Effects of the Death Penalty on Families of the Accused*

Robert H. Tillman and Michael L. Indergaard, *Pump and Dump: The Rancid Rules of the New Economy*

Mariana Valverde, *Law and Order: Images, Meanings, Myths*

Michael Welch, *Crimes of Power and States of Impunity: The U.S. Response to Terror*

Michael Welch, *Scapegoats of September 11th: Hate Crimes and State Crimes in the War on Terror*

Saundra D. Westervelt and Kimberly J. Cook, *Life after Death Row: Exonerees' Search for Community and Identity*

CPSIA information can be obtained
at www.ICGtesting.com
Printed in the USA
LVOW03s2237010318
568348LV00001B/104/P